PSYCHIATRY - THEORY, APPLICATIONS AND TREATMENTS

RATIONAL SUICIDE

IS IT POSSIBLE?

REFLECTIONS ON THE SUICIDE OF MARTIN MANLEY

PSYCHIATRY - THEORY, APPLICATIONS AND TREATMENTS

Additional books in this series can be found on Nova's website under the Series tab.

Additional e-books in this series can be found on Nova's website under the e-book tab.

RATIONAL SUICIDE

IS IT POSSIBLE?

REFLECTIONS ON THE SUICIDE OF MARTIN MANLEY

DAVID LESTER

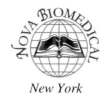

New York

For permission to use material from this book please contact us:
Telephone 631-231-7269; Fax 631-231-8175
Web Site: http://www.novapublishers.com

NOTICE TO THE READER

The Publisher has taken reasonable care in the preparation of this book, but makes no expressed or implied warranty of any kind and assumes no responsibility for any errors or omissions. No liability is assumed for incidental or consequential damages in connection with or arising out of information contained in this book. The Publisher shall not be liable for any special, consequential, or exemplary damages resulting, in whole or in part, from the readers' use of, or reliance upon, this material. Any parts of this book based on government reports are so indicated and copyright is claimed for those parts to the extent applicable to compilations of such works.

Independent verification should be sought for any data, advice or recommendations contained in this book. In addition, no responsibility is assumed by the publisher for any injury and/or damage to persons or property arising from any methods, products, instructions, ideas or otherwise contained in this publication.

This publication is designed to provide accurate and authoritative information with regard to the subject matter covered herein. It is sold with the clear understanding that the Publisher is not engaged in rendering legal or any other professional services. If legal or any other expert assistance is required, the services of a competent person should be sought. FROM A DECLARATION OF PARTICIPANTS JOINTLY ADOPTED BY A COMMITTEE OF THE AMERICAN BAR ASSOCIATION AND A COMMITTEE OF PUBLISHERS.

Additional color graphics may be available in the e-book version of this book.

Library of Congress Cataloging-in-Publication Data

ISBN: 978-1-62948-666-6

Library of Congress Control Number: 2013955543

Published by Nova Science Publishers, Inc. † New York

This book is dedicated to Martin Manley, a courageous man
Born 8-15-53, Died 8-15-13, Age 60

Contents

Preface

Martin Manley was a former sports star, journalist and blogger. He died by suicide on August 15th 2013 on his 60th birthday. The police in Overland Park, Kansas, found his body in the parking lot of the police station at 5 a.m. that Thursday morning. Martin had worked at the *Kansas City Star* for seven years, leaving the paper in February 2012 to start his own blog. He had written several books on sports statistics and is credited with creating the Efficiency Index used by the NBA.

Martin created a website at Yahoo (martinmanleylifeanddeath.com) and paid for five years to maintain it, in order to present his life's story to readers and explain the reasons for his decision to die by suicide. It always surprises me that, in this Internet age, and with presumably freedom of speech, such a website is disabled. Luckily, in this Internet age, there is usually a way to circumvent such intrusions. The material presented in this book comes from a mirror website www.zeroshare.info.

Other mirror sites are:

eulopedia.com/home_page.html
martinmanley.org
www.ussolutions.net/martin/backup/index-2.html
martinmanleylifeanddeath.com.nyud.net/home_page

Martin's sports website is www.sportsinreview.com/blog and his friends have set up a memorial website: www.martinmanleymemorial.blogspot.com/

The *Kansas City Star* announced his suicide in this way:

From The Kansas City Star,
August 16, 2013

Former Star Sports Statistics Editor, Blogger Commits Suicide at Overland Park Police Station

A former Kansas City Star sports statistics editor and blogger committed suicide early Thursday outside an Overland Park police station. Police found Martin

Manley's body about 5 a.m. Thursday in the parking lot of the station at 12400 Forest Ave.

"Martin was a terrific guy and a good employee," said Mike Fannin, editor and vice president of The Star. "This is a real shock, just an incredible tragedy. Our hearts and thoughts are with his family today."

Prior to his death, Manley detailed information about his life and suicide on a personal website. On the site, Manley referred to owning thousands of dollars-worth of gold and silver coins. Immediately following that reference were GPS coordinates for a spot inside the Overland Park Arboretum and Botanical Gardens. Police say they believe that statement is a hoax. They say his family told them that Manley had "gotten rid of" the coins prior to his suicide.

Manley killed himself on his 60th birthday. He had worked at The Star for seven years. He left The Star in February 2012 to start his own blog, Martin Manley's Sports in Review. Manley also had published several books on sports statistics and was credited with creating the NBA's Efficiency Index, which is still used by the league.

Star policy is not to write about suicides, except when they occur in public areas, as Manley's did.

The news media presented his suicide as motivated by dementia, a convenient assertion that the public could accept without feeling threatened. The truth is far from this. Some of us who study suicidal behavior believe that the decision to die by suicide can be a rational decision. We are in a minority, especially since the field of suicide studies is dominated by psychiatrists who believe that most of us are psychiatrically disturbed, let alone those who die by suicide.

My goal in this book is to present a defense of rational suicide and illustrate my defense with the essays written by Martin. Martin gave the world permission to use his essays on his website.[1]

Release of Rights

I, Martin Manley, being the creator and owner of all information on the site "MartinManleyLifeAndDeath.com", neither hold nor retain any claim or copyright on any part of this web-site. I do not grant these rights to any individual person or entity either in life or upon death. Rather I release all rights to this work – making it public domain. Anyone can do with it whatever they wish.

Before we look at Martin's essays, I will write on some general issues. First, I will discuss what we mean by rationality and irrationality. These words have many meanings, and some debates become confused because the debaters are using different definitions of the terms. Second, people often confuse illogical with irrational, and this issue needs to be clarified. Third, I have always thought that our deaths should be appropriate, but what does

---

[1] Martin wrote several essays that do not provide information about his motivates for choosing to die by suicide or his thoughts about it. I have not included those. They are available on his websites.

this mean? I will discuss several ways in which a death can be considered to be appropriate. Finally, in this introductory section, I have to address the issue of psychiatric disorder. In those states and nations which have passed legislation to permit assisted suicide, in which a physician is allowed to prescribe a lethal dose of a medication to an individual, an absence of psychiatric disorder is critical. I will discuss whether this is meaningful and whether it is fair, and in doing so I will deliver a strong attack on the field of psychiatry.

Let us begin our journey with a discussion of what it means to be rational.

Part 1: Introduction

Chapter 1

Can the Decision to Commit Suicide Be Rational?

Wilber (1987) argued that suicides interpret their experiences differently from nonsuicidal people. They fail to realize that there are several options open to them and, as a result, see suicide as the only way to deal with their intolerable circumstances. Their hopelessness makes their evaluation of their circumstances astigmatic. But, given their astigmatic perception of reality, their decision to commit suicide appears to be a logically valid deduction. Wilber, is, therefore, suggesting that the premises of the suicide are false, but that their argument is valid.

This issue is dealt with in detail by cognitive therapists who view the thinking patterns of all distressed people as irrational. Irrational thinking about events leads to pathological emotions and behavior. These ideas were originally formulated by Albert Ellis (1973) in his Rational-Emotive Therapy. Ellis described several common irrational thoughts that often underlie thinking, such as the idea that we should be thoroughly competent, adequate and achieving in all possible respects in order to consider ourselves worthwhile and the idea that certain people are bad, wicked and villainous and that they should be severely punished and blamed for their villainy. Burns (1980) has described more general irrational thinking patterns such as overgeneralizing (in which one negative event is seen as a never-ending pattern of negative events) and catastrophizing (seeing a negative event as the worst thing that could ever happen to you).

Although in America, defendants in a criminal trial are assumed to be innocent until proved to be guilty, in France defendants are presumed to be guilty and must prove their innocence. Therapists who view irrational thinking as the basis for pathological emotions and behavior take the French position. They place the burden of proof on the client whom they believe is thinking irrationally. If after your marriage breaks up, you say, "I will never find happiness with a lover," the cognitive therapist asks, "Where is the proof that you will never find happiness with a lover?" You are required to prove your belief. The therapist, who obviously is implying the opposite, is not required to prove his or her belief. I have known people who have never found someone to love them and who have never been in a long-term happy relationship. Some are in their sixties and, probably, never will find anyone. Had they made those statements, labeled irrational by Ellis, they would in fact have been correct.

Furthermore, although logicians define inductive arguments as those in which the premises provide some support, but not absolute support, for a conclusion, they do not define the word "some." Suppose I have been rejected by one lover, two, or perhaps three. How many must reject me to meet the criterion for "some support" for the inductive generalization? Conclusions are often judged to be irrational by cognitive therapists because the person has over-generalized, but cognitive therapists, like logicians, do not propose how many occurrences permit generalization.

The fact that inductive reasoning may sometimes lead to false conclusions is no argument against it. The possibility of false conclusions is inherent in the definition of inductive reasoning but, sometimes, it is the only form of reasoning available to us.

Is Suicide the Result of a Decision?

Before examining whether a decision to commit suicide can be rational, it is worthwhile considering whether suicide is the result of a decision. For example, if a schizophrenic hears a voice commanding him to jump off a building and fly and if he obeys, his resulting death is not the result of a reasoned decision. In this context, Goldstein's (1940) strict criteria for judging a death to be suicidal are relevant. Goldstein said that the person must have a mature concept of death and must consciously choose death. Only suicidal deaths which meet these criteria may be viewed as decisions.[1]

The more determinants researchers identify for a behavior, the less easy it is to claim that the behavior was a result of a decision. If schizophrenia is really the result of a genetically-programmed defect in the dopamine and norepinephrine neurotransmitters in the brain, then it makes little sense to talk about a decision to be schizophrenic. Similarly, if suicide can be shown to have biochemical and early event precursors, then the behavior appears to be more determined and less of a decision. However, it has been impossible so far to identify *necessary* and *sufficient* determinants for suicidal behavior.

Despite these caveats, suicidal individuals usually feel subjectively that they are making a decision, and those taking away our right to die by suicide view it as a decision (albeit an irrational decision). Therefore, asking whether the decision can be rational remains reasonable.

Can Psychiatrically Disturbed People Have Rational Premises?

This issue is so important in the discussion of rational suicide that it demands its own chapter (Chapter 4). Here I will simply note that some writers on this topic have used the psychiatric disturbance of most suicides as evidence that they could not have been thinking rationally. Pretzel (1968), for example, noted that we often endorse four types of suicide as rational: (i) suicides carried out for some cause (such as martyrdom), (ii) suicide as a reaction

---

[1] Menninger (1938) had a much broader definition of suicide that included partial and unconsciously motivated self-destructive behavior.

to a lingering, painful, and incurable illness, (iii) suicide where the individual is not receiving any pleasure from life, and (iv) love-pact suicides. Pretzel selected a case study of each of these types of suicide and demonstrated some degree of psychiatric disturbance in the people involved. He concluded that in each case there were psychopathological factors at work in the motivation of the suicide and, therefore, that the suicide was irrational. His approach was biased, of course, because he could have selected a non-disturbed case for each type of suicide since not all suicides are demonstrably disturbed. Although some psychiatrists have found almost all suicides to be psychiatrically disturbed in retrospect (e.g., Robins, 1981), not all psychiatrists agree, and estimates of the percentage of the psychiatrically disturbed in samples of suicides range from 5 to 94 percent (Temoche, et al., 1964).

I will explore this issue in greater detail later in Chapter 4.

Rationality and the Statistical Rarity of Suicide

The statistical rarity of suicide means that only a very small proportion of people experiencing any trauma kill themselves. For example, even among those diagnosed with an affective disorder or who have attempted suicide, only about 15 percent of their deaths are from suicide. The statistical rarity of suicide means that the precipitating conditions can never be considered necessary or sufficient. This fact leads many observers to judge suicide to be irrational.

Others, however, may view suicide committed as a result of particular precipitants as rational. This typically means that the observer thinks that he or she might also have committed suicide under such circumstances. If we think that we might kill ourselves if we were dying from cancer, then suicide under those circumstances would be judged to be rational. If we would never immolate ourselves on the steps of the Capitol Building in Washington, DC, in order to bring peace to the world, then we would probably view such suicides as irrational. The judgment of suicide as rational on this basis is an example of the *subjective definition of normality*.

Nevertheless, when we feel that a suicide is precipitated by sufficient stressors, we may view the suicide as *understandable*, and Margolis (1975), for example, equates *understandable* with *justified*. In recent years, suicide committed by people dying from painful incurable cancers or AIDS-related infections has been widely viewed as rational.

Do Unconscious Forces Make Suicide Irrational?

If you do not believe in the Freudian (psychoanalytic) or another form of the unconscious (Jungian or simply cognitive unawareness), then this is not an issue for deciding whether a decision is motivated in part by unconscious desires, thoughts and emotions. However, I believe in the existence of a Freudian unconscious, having become aware of its operation in my own life and of the usefulness of the concept for explaining human behavior, although I follow the version of theory presented by an Austrian psychoanalyst, Walter Toman (1960).

Unconscious motivations, in all likelihood, play a role in all of our decisions. For example, most of us are not fully aware of why we fell in love with those we loved; nor why we married them. Yet those decisions are not typically viewed as irrational.[2] Even those of our decisions that we believe to be fully rational may have unconscious determinants. Thus, if we do not call into question the irrationality of the majority of our decisions, why should we do so for the decision to die by suicide and, as a consequence, see it as appropriate to force someone into a psychiatric hospital (which should better be called a prison) in order to prevent them from carrying out this act.

Antoon Leenaars (1986) has documented the existence of unconscious determinants in suicide notes. Since the Freudian unconscious is typically viewed as using irrational thinking patterns, suicide motivated by unconscious forces may appear to be irrational. Antoon Leenaars and I have edited a book on the role of the unconscious in the decision to die by suicide. (Leenaars & Lester, 1996).

Further Definitions of Rationality?

As we can see, the word rational is used in many ways, and it is important to distinguish the various meanings and explore the implications of each for viewing suicide as rational or irrational. We have already discussed rationality viewed from the viewpoint of truth, necessary and sufficient causes, psychiatric disorder, statistical rarity, and unconscious motivation. Other viewpoints are possible.

Empirical Judgments of Rationality

We might look at the outcome of the suicidal action as a basis for deciding whether the suicidal action was rational or not. For example, if the suicidal action changes the person's life for the better, perhaps it was a rational action? Certainly, as Nietzsche is commonly quoted as saying, the thought of suicide helps many people through a crisis. An individual can say that, if things get worse, he can always kill himself, a thought that gives him enough energy and motivation to live another day during which time, perhaps, the strength of the suicidal impulse decreases. To take another example, one patient who, when assured that no one would interfere if she tried to kill herself, decided not to do so since now she felt back in charge of her life.

Attempted suicides are often pleased with the changes in interpersonal relationships brought about by their suicide attempt. But can we say that the completed suicide ever changes their life for the better? This of course depends on how one evaluates the life which the suicide is leading relative to death. Was death worse than life in a concentration camp under the Nazis? Surprisingly, few inmates of those camps committed suicide, although Lester (2005) has shown that previous estimates of very low suicide rates were erroneous.[3] Perhaps they viewed life as better. Yet many did commit suicide, directly or indirectly, and so perhaps they viewed death as better. The judgment made by the prisoners was subjective.

---

[2] I have heard it claimed that falling in love is a time-limited psychiatrically disturbed state of mind, and that no decisions should be made while in that state of mind! I also remember a Bishop once telling an interviewer that he would die knowing that he made at least one person happy When the interviewer asked who, the Bishop replied, "The woman I didn't marry!"

[3] His estimates suggest that the suicide rate could have been as high as 25,000 per 100,000 per year.

Rational or Autonomous

Beauchamp and Childress (1979) have noted that suicide can be an autonomous act by a person (that is, an act that is freely chosen[4]), and suicide by an autonomous individual which also meets utilitarian criteria (maximizing good and minimizing harm) is possible. Hauerwas (1981) felt that autonomous individuals could commit rational suicide, although he found such suicides not to be morally justified.

Can suicide be the action of an autonomous individual? The right of people to refuse extraordinary medical treatment has been viewed as acceptable by the federal courts in America, and suicide differs from this only in the activity (versus the passivity) of the behavior. Suicide is not illegal in any American state and so, at least by implication, individuals have the right to commit suicide.

Rational Versus Emotional

Hauerwas (1981) contrasted rational suicide (which he defined as cool and unemotional) with (by implication) emotional and impulsive suicide. He gave the Stoics of ancient Greece as examples of rational suicide using these criteria. Can suicide ever be the action of a cool and unemotional person?

Such suicides probably exist, although we would need neutral observers to be present to witness the death in order to be sure. Some of the suicides by terminally-ill individuals probably meet this criterion. As far as we can tell, Freud's physician-assisted suicide, for which he had made arrangements many years earlier, may well have met this criterion.

Economic Views of Suicide

Can suicide be rational using the criteria of economists? Yeh and Lester (1987) presented a cost-benefit analysis of suicide in which the individual is assumed to weigh the costs and benefits of suicide as a strategy as compared to the costs and benefits of other alternatives. Clarke and Lester (1989) have also presented such an analysis. Thus, if these analyses have merit, it may be that suicide maximizes utility.

Yang and Lester (2006) reviewed several economic theories of suicide which conceptualize suicide as a rational act, including the cost-benefit analysis mentioned above, a demand-and-supply model, a lifetime utility maximization model, a labor-force analogy model, an investment under uncertainty mode, and a signaling game.

In psychoanalytic theory, desires, both conscious and unconscious, motivate all behavior, and all behavior is a compromise of conflicting desires. Thus, choices in this perspective can always be seen as maximizing psychological utility. The fact that some of the desires may be unconscious has no relevance to this criterion.

---

[4] The definition of autonomous is a person or entity that is self-controlling and not governed by outside forces.

Does the Decision to Commit Suicide Follow Rational Laws?

Lester (1996-1997) presented students with scenarios in which they had AIDS and had differing probabilities of surviving for one year and different levels of pain. When asked to estimate the probability that they would commit suicide under these circumstances, their estimate was higher the more pain and the greater the chance of dying within a year from AIDS. The results made sense – this is what one would expect rational people to decide.

Lester (2003) suggested that decisions to commit suicide that follow meaningful psychological principles can be considered to be rational. Whereas many commentators assert that depressed people cannot make a rational decision to commit suicide *because* they are depressed, Lester argued that it is more rational for depressed people to commit suicide than for happy people to commit suicide.

Making a Rational Decision to Commit Suicide

Lester (2003) laid out a process by which individuals could make a rational decision to commit suicide.

1. First, individuals should list all of their current problems. Are you depressed, lonely, an alcoholic, etc?
2. Lester suggested that individuals should follow Greenwald's (1973) system of Direct Decision Therapy and consider whether they made a decision to have this state or problem. Did you decide to be depressed, for example? When and under what circumstances? Greenwald considered all problems to be the product, at least in part, of a decision made by the individual at an earlier time in life. When the context in which the decision was made is discovered, then the decision does not appear to be as irrational or inappropriate as one might think.
3. If the individuals are considering suicide at the present time, what is it about the problems that lead them to consider this? Is it the physical pain, the limitations on your lifestyle, the financial burden to your family, etc?
4. Taking each of these features in turn, suicide is clearly one option. What are other options? If you are concerned about the burden on others who may have to disrupt their life in order to take care of you, are there other alternatives, such as relatives for whom it would not as much a burden, a home health-care aide who could come to perform some of the chores, or a hospice to go to until death?

Each option, suicide and the alternatives, have costs and benefits. In Direct Decision Therapy, Greenwald has his clients specify these costs and benefits for each alternative course of action. Lester suggested getting those involved in your life to collaborate on this task and to keep careful written notes that can be referred to when needed.

The involvement of significant others is crucial here. You may worry about the financial burden on your loved-ones and on leaving them some inheritance, but they may not be concerned about this at all. They may choose to have you in their lives for a longer time and forego any inheritance. You may worry that they cannot cope with the nursing care you will need, but they may view this as manageable.

5. If, after going through all of these steps, you choose to commit suicide, it is important that your significant others have some input. They need to express their point of view and listen to yours, and, if possible, a mutually agreed-upon decision made. But, in the end, it is your life and your decision.

6. Finally, Lester noted that decisions are not necessarily final. You can change your mind. You can choose to undergo chemotherapy for your cancer and, after a while, change your mind. You can decide to commit suicide, but change this decision as you make the preparatory steps.

An Example

A good example of this process comes from the Netherlands, reported by René Diekstra (1995). Mr. L had cancer and was given no more than six months to live. He was a retired civil servant, a stubborn man with a defeatist attitude toward life. His wife was informed of his prognosis first and communicated this to her husband, after which he declared that he wished to end his life with medications. He felt that his life was useless, and he feared dependence on physicians, burdening his wife with nursing, and the degeneration of his body.

One of his sons was a physician, but he refused to become involved with his father's decision. Mr. L's general practitioner refused to provide medications but said that he would withhold treatment if, for example, Mr. L caught pneumonia. The other family members did not object to Mr. L's suicide, but Mr. L's wife thought that it was too soon for him to die. Their relationship was still rewarding, and she saw that her husband could still enjoy some aspects of living, at least for a while. She did not want him to die in pain from the cancer, but she also feared that her husband might try to kill himself by other, more violent methods if he was not provided with medication, a situation that she would find traumatic.

At Diekstra's suggestion, Mr. L's wife told her husband that she thought it was too early for him to die and that she would miss him if he died at that moment. He was pleased to hear this and glad that he was still needed. He agreed to postpone the decision, but he wanted assurance that he would be given the medication when the appropriate time arrived. He was given this assurance, and he lived for two more months.

Diekstra noted that, apart from simply providing the man with the necessary medication for suicide, he acknowledged the acceptability of Mr. L's request and mobilized communication within the family, getting the wife and the children involved. Mr. L came to feel less anxious and agitated, and he was able to participate more constructively in the life of his family for his final two months of life. The process improved the quality of life for both Mr. L and his family.

Diekstra pointed out that "assisted suicide" means more than just providing the medications necessary for death. It should also involve providing technical information on the means for committing suicide, removal of obstacles such as getting the person released from an institution, giving advice on precautions and actions (such as making a will), and remaining with the person until the very end. We might add that it should also involve the counseling of both the client and the significant others by a counselor who is sensitized to the issues involved.

Another excellent example of this process is provided by Roman (1980) who documented her decision to stop chemotherapy for cancer and to commit suicide. She made the decision along with her husband and also involved her friends and relatives in the process (see Chapter 32).

Discussion

What I have tried to accomplish so far in this chapter is to present a set of definitions to clarify the question of whether suicide can be logical or rational. Irrationality can refer to (1) the degree of psychiatric disturbance of the individual, (2) the statistical rarity of a behavior, (3) whether there are unconscious processes motivating the behavior, at least in part, (4) whether the behavior improved the state of the person, (5) whether the behavior was that of an autonomous individual, (6) whether the decision was affected by emotional states, (7) whether the behavior maximized utility, and (8) whether we find the reasons for the behavior to be acceptable. Of course, some of these criteria might be judged more salient to the decision to commit suicide than others.

Obviously suicide can be irrational. The critical question, therefore, is whether suicide can ever be rational. Since we are rarely around the individual who is about to commit suicide and since there are few standardized psychological tests to measure the variables involved in the criteria listed above, the question may be unanswerable. However, some investigators do find some suicides to be free of psychiatric illness, and some suicides meet the criteria for being autonomous individuals. Occasional suicides do seem to improve the state of the person and maximize utility (both for the suicide and the society). And, unless one thinks that suicide is never acceptable, most of us could find acceptable reasons for suicide. However, suicide is always statistically rare and, if one accepts the existence of the unconscious, is probably always motivated in part by unconscious forces.

Finally, there may be some suicides for whom their premises are true or, at least, not demonstrably false, and whose reasoning is valid and free from the many kinds of fallacies which logicians have described (Engel, 1986), and this might be most easily demonstrated by those suicides who meet the economists criteria for maximizing utility.

I studied the lives of thirty suicides sufficiently interesting and famous for biographies and autobiographies to have been published (Lester, 1991). Do any of those lives fit the criteria above? The presence of psychological disturbance in many of the suicides makes it difficult to be sure without an interview with the person prior to their death to explore whether some of the criteria listed above could be met. However, the physician-assisted suicide of Sigmund Freud, who was in the end stages of a painful cancer (Gay, 1988), came closest to meeting many of the criteria.

Chapter 2

The Logic of Suicidal Individuals

Logic may be defined as the study of the laws of thought or the study of reasoning, but such a definition fails to distinguish logic from psychology. Psychology describes the ways in which people actually reason. In contrast, logic sets standards for the ways in which people ought to reason if they wished to reason well. Logic evaluates the quality of the reasoning.

Sentences are said to be cognitive when they are used to express or assert something which may be true or false (Baum, 1974). The thought conveyed by a cognitive sentence is called a statement or proposition. The truth or falsity of a statement may depend upon the truth or falsity of related statements – commonly called supported statements. Other statements can stand on their own – self-supporting statements. The burden of proof for a statement being self-supporting falls on those who consider it to be false. Two statements may be consistent (it is possible for both to be true at the same time) or inconsistent (it is impossible for both of them to be true at the same time). An argument is a set of statements which is such that one of them (the conclusion) is implied or supported by the others (the premises).

There are two critical evaluations in logic. Validity refers to arguments of which, if the premises are true, then the conclusion must also be true. Truth refers to whether the premises or the conclusions are true or false. A valid deductive argument is one where, if the premises are true, then the conclusion must be true. An argument whose premises provide some support, but not absolute support for the conclusion, is called an inductive argument.

Thus, analysis of the logical of suicide entails first describing the reasoning engaged in by the suicidal person, evaluating the validity of the reasoning, and finally evaluating the truth of the premises and conclusion. Arguments that are both true and valid may be called sound.

Shneidman's Views on the Logic of Suicide

Shneidman (1970) noted that the formal logic of suicidal reasoning is not as interesting as the actual style of reasoning used by the individual, what he termed *concludifying*, that is, how the individual reaches conclusions, thinks, reasons and infers. Shneidman called the individual's style of concludifying his or her *idio-logic*. Idio-logic includes both the aspects of reasoning which might be subsumed under the traditional fallacies of reasoning, as well as the cognitive maneuvers which describe the cognitive style of the individual. In addition, Shneidman analyzed the *contra-logic* of the individual, that is, the private epistemological and metaphysical view of the universe inferred from the idio-logic. Finally, there are overt and covert aspects of personality which are related to and reflective of the individual's style of thinking, his or her *psycho-logic*. In this chapter, I am concerned only with the idio-logical of the suicidal individual.

Logic Versus Psychologic

In several papers, Shneidman made a distinction between pure logic and the logic that ordinary people use, psychologic. As an example of this, Shneidman (1982a) considered the use of the word "therefore." He argued that people use the word in ways that do not imply "always" or "under all circumstances". Shneidman suggested that the mind does not syllogize in a logical sense, but rather concludifies (comes to conclusions) in a psycho-logical sense. "Therefore, I must commit suicide" may mean a variety of things to the individual, such as I may commit suicide, I ought to commit suicide, I should commit suicide, I might commit suicide, I shall commit suicide, and I must commit suicide. The thought may refer to the present time or the future. It may refer to all circumstances or only to some circumstances. Shneidman warned psychotherapists to be aware of this flexible usage of the word "therefore" and to take care to understand precisely what the client means, rather than simply assuming that the client is using the word in a formal logic sense. Shneidman noted that the use of the word "therefore" by people is closer to the Persian logic of centuries ago which included the temporal dimension of ubiquity versus occasionality as well as a dimension of necessity or certainty versus probability.

Fallacies

Shneidman and Farberow (1970) suggested one fallacy that suicidal individuals may make in their reasoning. Although they called this type of reasoning *catalogic*, since it destroys the reasoner, they also called it, more accurately, a *psychosemantic fallacy*. They suggested that some suicidal individuals confuse the self as experienced by themselves with the self as experienced by others. If the suicidal individual reasons, "If a person kills himself, he gets attention; I will kill myself, therefore I will get attention," the "I" that kills is the self as experienced by the self while the "I" that gets attention is the self as experienced by others. This fallacy is called by logicians the fallacy of equivocation (Engel, 1986). Shneidman and Farberow noted that this fallacy is avoided if the suicidal individual believes in a life after death in which case he or she will be able to watch the reaction of others.

Shneidman (1970) gave other examples of fallacies in suicidal thinking. One very brief suicide note read as follows: "I love everybody but my darling wife has killed me." Shneidman noted the suppressed premise – therefore, I kill myself. The man's logic is: If X loves Y and Y kills X, then X must kill X. Once this suppressed premise is added to the argument, then the fallacy of equivocation in the use of the word *kill* is apparent. Kill is used figuratively in the overt premise to mean betray or violated, while in the suppressed premise it is used literally.

The Idio-Logic of Cesare Pavese

Shniedman (1982b) examined the diary of Cesare Pavese, the Italian writer who killed himself in 1950, and identified two styles of thinking in Pavese.

1. A style of combining opposites, juxtaposing assertions with denials and contradictory ideas. For example, "The richness of life lies in memories we have forgotten" (February 13, 1944) or "The unique event which you find so exciting can only have its full value if it has never taken place" (February 13, 1945).
2. A constricting style of thinking so that he limited his options to a narrow few. For example, "To choose a hardship for ourselves is our only defense against that hardship....This is how we can disarm the power of suffering, make it our own creation, our own choice; submit to it" (November 10, 1938). Pavese perceives only one option here, whereas in fact there are many strategies open to him.

In addition, Shneidman observed a different form of illogical reasoning. "If I were dead, she would go on living laughing, trying her luck. But she has thrown me over and still does all those things. Therefore, I am as dead" (February 25, 1938). "If A, then B" does not imply "If B, then A." This error in propositional logic is commonly called *affirming the consequent* (or consequence). "If I drop objects, they fall to the ground" does not imply. "This object fell to the ground (imagine a meteor), therefore I dropped it." The word "as" in the phrase "I am as dead" possibly makes Pavese's argument literary rather than (il)logical, but using such phrasing may well have shaped Pavese's reasoning.

Shneidman noted that Pavese's suicide was not due to faulty logic. Rather Pavese's style of thinking and reasoning directly predisposed him to make a suicidal decision when the stress he felt was great.

Conclusion

It would appear that, unless a person has grossly psychotic thought patterns, then the logic of suicidal individuals is fine. It is their premises or assumptions that critics call into question.

Chapter 3

Can Suicide be an Appropriate Death?

When psychologists consider the question of what is a good death, they talk about an "appropriate" death rather than a "good" death. A good death is what "euthanasia" means literally, but the term euthanasia now has acquired a variety of connotations which can upset people -- for example, it has become associated with "mercy killing," that is, killing someone to end their misery, not necessarily with their permission or agreement.

Accordingly, this chapter will address whether suicide can be an appropriate death. How might we define this concept?[1]

Weisman and Hackett

Although the literature is not very extensive, there are some scholars who have written about the concept of an appropriate death (or dying). In 1961, Avery Weisman and Thomas Hackett wrote an article that brought the concept to the attention of psychiatrists. Weisman and Hackett noted that some of their patients knew, correctly as it turned out, the exact time when they were going to die, and yet faced their impending death without conflict, depression, suicidal ideation or panic. They did not act like those hexed into death by suggestion (sometimes called "voodoo death"), after which they become hopeless and helpless. On the contrary, Weisman and Hackett's patients knew that death was inevitable, and they desired it. For these patients, death was faced peacefully, calmly, and without apparent worry. After reflecting on their experiences with these patients, Weisman and Hackett proposed four specific criteria for a death (or a dying process) to be considered appropriate.

1. Most importantly, death must be seen as an event that reduces the conflict in your life or that is a solution to problems you are facing. (Alternatively, there may be few conflicts or problems in your life.)

---

[1] The following list is not exhaustive -- I am sure that other definitions can be proposed. I will present you with some possible definitions simply to stimulate your thinking on the issue.

2. Death must be seen as being compatible with your conscience -- for example, you do not view your death as a cowardly act or as a sin.
3. There must be a continuity of important relationships as you die (for example, dying with your loved ones beside you), or there must be some prospect of the relationships being restored (for example, being reunited with loved ones after you die).
4. Finally, you must sincerely desire death.

Because Weisman and Hackett's criteria for an appropriate death were originally proposed only for deaths from natural causes, they did not include suicide as a possible type of appropriate death. However, a suicidal death can meet each of these four criteria and, therefore, be an appropriate death. You may be facing few problems, or your death from suicide would reduce conflict in your life (criterion 1). Your moral philosophy may enable you to see suicide as an acceptable act (criterion 2). You may expect to be reunited with loved ones after your suicide (criterion 3), and you probably do sincerely desire death (criterion 4).

The Different Kinds of Death

Richard Kalish (1985) has identified four types of death -- physical, psychological, social and anthropological -- and his classification suggests another criterion for a death to be appropriate. Let me first define his terms.

Biological death is when your organs cease to function, and *clinical death* is when your organism as a whole ceases to function. These two forms of death constitute *physical death*. Biological and clinical death need not coincide in time. For example, it is possible for your organs to keep functioning after your brain has been removed from the body. In this situation, you are clinically dead but biologically alive. In fact, this is what happens when organs are removed from a person who has recently died so that they may be transplanted into others who need them.

You are *psychologically dead* when you cease to be aware of your own self and of your own existence. You do not know who you are nor that you even exist. A person in a coma is presumed to be psychologically dead.

Social death occurs when you accept the notion that, for all practical intents and purposes, you are dead, and you act as if you are dead. In cases of voodoo death, if you believe that you have been hexed and expect to die in a few days, you prepare for death. You may refuse nourishment and lay down in expectation of death. In this situation, you remain conscious, and so you are not yet psychologically dead, and you are certainly not physically dead.

Social death may also be defined from the point of view of friends and relatives. In this situation, you are socially dead when the people who know you act as if you no longer exist. For example, an elderly relative may be put in a home and forgotten, and the family acts as if she no longer exists. The relatives of a hexed individual may start grieving and preparing for the funeral.

The final kind of death, *anthropological death*, occurs when you are cut off from the entire community, rather than merely your relatives, and treated as if you no longer exist. The Orthodox Jew who marries a Gentile is anthropologically dead to the Orthodox community.

The Orthodox community and the person's family mourn for him just as if he were physically dead.

Kalish's four types of death provide a possible criterion for an appropriate death. These four kinds of death can occur at different times in your life. For example, an elderly parent may be put in a nursing home and forgotten about (social death), later fall seriously ill and become so senile that she loses awareness of who she is (psychological death), and even later finally succumb to her illness (physical death). In some families, a person may be mourned on several occasions.

A death could be considered appropriate when all four of these different kinds of death coincide in time. When they occur at different times, ethical and logistical issues are often raised. For example, when a person is in a coma, the issue of whether or when life support systems should be turned off may be raised. Thus, a person who falls into a coma (psychological death) and physically dies much later could be viewed as having an inappropriate death. The person who is placed in a nursing home and forgotten (social death) does not die an appropriate death. Using this criterion, suicide could be an appropriate death since all four kinds of death can occur at the same time in a suicidal death.

The Role of Individuals in Their Own Death

Some existentialists believe that death is appropriate only when you play a role in it. In other words, a person struck down by chance factors, such as lightning, would not have died an appropriate death. Obviously, suicides play a major role in their own death. When discussing the death by suicide of one of his psychiatric patients, Ludwig Binswanger (1958), an existential psychiatrist, believed that only in her manner of death did she "fully exist." For Binswanger, we exist authentically only when we resolve situations decisively by our actions. Binswanger's patient, whom he called Ellen West, was labeled as psychiatrically disturbed for most of her life. She was hospitalized on several occasions. Her symptoms dominated her life and restricted her opportunities for growth. In her decision to kill herself, she seemed to be making a choice, and for once she was not overwhelmed by her symptoms or the conflicts underlying her psychopathology. Her suicidal act was authentic.

In this regard, it is interesting to note that one of the many Japanese words for suicide is *jiketsu* which means self-determination (Rankin, 2011).

Physical Integrity in Death

Some people feel that a "natural" death is a good death because in a natural death, the body is physically intact and retains its physical integrity. For example, when a person commits suicide by shooting herself or a murder victim is stabbed to death, the body's physical integrity is lost, and the death may be considered inappropriate.[2] From this point of view, the death of someone whose life has been prolonged by the use of transplants and

---

[2] Edwin Shneidman has asserted that he found the intrusion of a lethal virus into his body no more "natural" than the intrusion of a bullet!

medical intrusions into the body cannot be appropriate. Only a death from natural causes without medical intrusion may be viewed as appropriate. Suicide could be appropriate under this criterion if a suitable method is used, such as an overdose of sleeping pills for, in this case, the physiological damage to the body is minimal (and perhaps less than is the case in death from such illnesses as cancer).

Consistency in Lifestyle

If I were to ask you how you would like to die, your response will reflect something about yourself, your personality and your fears, but it may also reflect your lifestyle, a lifestyle which has developed as a result of your inherited tendencies, experiences, personality, successes and failures. People will typically choose a death that fits with their lifestyle.

The passive person may choose to die from a disease or even at the hands of another. The aggressive person may choose to die in a fight or in war. The self-destructive person may commit suicide.

A person's death may be appropriate, therefore, if he dies in a way that is consistent with his or her lifestyle. For example, Ernest Hemingway's suicide by a firearm in the face of growing medical and psychiatric illness was consistent with the death-defying lifestyle he had cultivated during his lifetime. Hemingway ran with the bulls in Spain, hunted big game in Africa and sought to be in the front lines with the soldiers in Europe during the Second World War. He risked his life in all kinds of situations. It would be hard to imagine Hemingway dying as a shrunken old man, drooling in a corner of a locked ward in a mental hospital.

Suicide could be viewed as appropriate, then, if it is consistent with the person's lifestyle.

The Timing of Death

Edwin Shneidman (1967) suggested that the timing of our death was an important consideration in defining an appropriate death. Shneidman felt that people are sometimes able to discern that, after a given point, any further life would be a defeat or a pointless repetition. There may be points in time when death seems to be the right thing. For example, the Japanese novelist Yukio Mishima placed great importance on his physical appearance and on his skill as a writer. In 1970, at the age of 45, he thought that he had peaked and that his life from then on would decline. He no longer had confidence in his body or in his writing ability. Mishima killed himself by seppuku rather than face what to him would have been the shame of defeat.

At certain times in your life, a point may come when death would be appropriate and would complete your life's path (perhaps your life's work). Such a death might even heighten your significance by making your memory more treasured by your family or by posterity. Suicide could be consistent with this criterion.

Comment

The concept of an appropriate death is an important one, and these different criteria are relevant for the life and death of all individuals. Sometimes our lives seem to be full of forces and events over which we have no control. Powerful others, fate and chance events have a great impact on our lives. It can, therefore, be satisfying and empowering to exert some control over one of the more important events of our life -- the leaving of it.

Each of you should determine what an appropriate death is for you. Does one or more of the definitions above make sense for your death? If not, what other definition would you propose?

Included in the responsibilities of counselors, psychotherapists and doctors, who strive to help people improve their lives, should be the goal of helping patients to die an appropriate death. To do this, the counselor must first be aware of the alternative concepts for an appropriate death, and then must identify what the client believes. If death in one particular manner is more appropriate for a client than death in another manner, then perhaps it is the counselor's duty to allow and to facilitate the client to die in that way. Finally, it is not right to impose our definition of an appropriate death on others. What is right for me is not necessarily right for you.

By some definitions, suicide can be an appropriate death, and suicide can also be a rational death. Can it then be a good death? If these are our criteria, the answer is yes, and that is why I have written a book on the topic, *Fixin' to Die: A Compassionate Guide to Committing Suicide or Staying Alive* (Lester, 2003).

Chapter 4

The Issue of Psychiatric Disorder

In this chapter, I will discuss the critical issue of whether the presence of a psychiatric disorder in individuals precludes them from making rational decisions. In doing so, I will present a strong critique of the field of psychiatry which, in my opinion (and that of others such as Thomas Szasz [1974]) has departed from the tenets of good scientific theory and even those tenets of the model on which it is based (the scientific study of medical diseases). I will present my argument as a series of *objections*.

Objection 1: The Diagnostic System

To introduce you to my major objection, let us assume you have a headache and a fever. You go to your family physician, and he tells you that you have a disease called headache-fever, or HF for short. What would you do? You'd run as fast as you could out of his or her office and look for a good doctor. Medical illnesses are based on causes. What is causing your fever? What is causing your headache? Is it caused by a virus or bacteria? If so, which ones? Lyme's disease or swine flu? Is it because of a brain tumor and, if so, is it malignant or benign?

Psychiatric disorders or mental illnesses are not defined by causes. They are defined by clusters of symptoms. Let us say you are depressed. Maybe it is because you do not have enough serotonin in certain regions of the brain. Maybe you have suppressed and repressed anger felt toward significant others in your life so that you are no longer conscious of the anger (a Freudian, psychoanalytic view). Maybe it is because you have learned from you life's experiences that you cannot get of the traps in which you find yourself (learned helplessness). Maybe it is because that are not enough rewards (positive reinforcers) in your life, either because you are in unrewarding relationships and employment or because you lack the skills to obtain rewards from others (a learning theory perspective).

Maybe it is simply the melancholia that is part of all of our lives (Wilson, 2008)? Where is it ordained that we deserve to be happy? A friend of mine from our childhood days lost his wife to brain cancer when they were in their early 50s, leaving him with their two adolescent children. He grieved, but his physician thought that he was depressed and prescribed him Prozac, gradually increasing the dose to three times the recommended amount, a dose so high that that his doctor had to wean him off it gradually when he realized that it had not helped his grief. He was NOT psychiatrically ill. He was grieving, and it takes each of us a different amount of time to get over such a loss. Today, twenty years later, he is fine, and involved in a new relationship and enjoying life. Eric Wilson's book argues that melancholy is a normal state of humans from time to time, and even for long periods of time. Melancholy is *not* a disease.

If your depression is blocked anger, then a psychiatric pill is a stupid treatment. Help the person recognize and deal with his or her anger. If the depression is learned helplessness, then teach them coping skills so that they do not feel helpless. If I were in charge of the National Institute of Mental Health, I would abandon the current system and put out a "call for proposals" for a new diagnostic system based on causes.

Don't be fooled by the new revision of the *Diagnostic and Statistical Manual* (DSM). Version 5 has now been published, and it is not an improvement. For example, on pages 160-161, it lists the criteria for diagnosing a *major depressive disorder*. There is a list of 9 symptoms that must be present for at least two weeks. Here is an abbreviated version of each symptom: (i) depressed mood most of the day, (ii) diminished interest in all activities, (iii) significant weight loss (without dieting) or weight gain, (iv) insomnia or hypersomnia, (v) psychomotor agitation or retardation, (vi) fatigue or loss of energy, (vii) feelings of worthlessness, (viii) diminished ability to think or concentrate, and (ix) recurrent thoughts of death and suicide. DSM-5 does discuss associated features, prevalence, development and course, risk and prognostic factors, culture-related diagnostic issues, gender-related diagnostic issues, suicide risk, functional consequences of major depressive disorder, differential diagnosis, and comorbity. But the criteria for this disease, disorders, or illness (call it what you will) still do not involve *causes*!

Part of the motivation for revising the DSM is that psychiatrists cannot agree on which "illness" patients have. Using an older version of the DSM, Beck and his colleagues (1962) found that four psychiatrists, individually interviewing the same psychiatric patients, agreed only 54% of the time for the specific diagnosis and only 70% for the major category (schizophrenia, affective disorder, anxiety disorder, personality disorder, etcetera). In another study of the older version of the DSM, Sandifer and his colleagues had psychiatrists in three cities view tape-recorded interviews of psychiatric patients. In North Carolina, the patients were more often labeled as having neurotic disorders, In Glasgow, Scotland, the same patients were more often labeled as having personality disorders, and in London (England) the patients were more often labeled as having bipolar affective disorder (manic-depressive disorder)!

There have been three modern critiques of the current psychiatric system. Robert Whitaker's *Anatomy of an epidemic: Magic bullets, psychiatric drugs, and the astonishing rise of mental illness in America*, Irving Kirsch's *The Emperor's new drugs: Exploding the antidepressant myth*, and Daniel Carlat's *Unhinged: The trouble with psychiatry*. These books were favorably reviewed by Marcia Angell, a former editor of *The New England Journal of Medicine,* a prestigious scholarly medical journal, in *The New York Review of Books* (June 23 and July 14, 2012). Whitaker, for example, argues forcefully that (i) there is no sound evidence that psychiatric disorders have a physiological basis, (ii) psychiatric medications create chemical imbalances in the brain that persist even when patients stop taking the medications and that cause the brain to behave abnormally, and (iii) patients given placebos (particularly those that create harmless but noticeable side-effects [the so-called active placebos]) improve as much as patients given psychiatric medications. Loren Mosher, a prominent psychiatrist, resigned from the American Psychiatric Association back in 1998, accusing the association of selling out to the pharmaceutical industry that markets psychiatric medications.[1]

I am not arguing here that these writers who have attacked the psychiatric model are one hundred percent correct. I am saying that readers should be aware that there are strong voices (besides mine) arguing that the psychiatric model is seriously flawed and needs drastic revision.

One final comment here. If you decide to kill yourself and if you want to use a medication, you will have problems getting prescriptions in order to obtain sufficient medication. Who will find it most easy to accumulate the lethal overdose? Psychiatrists and physicians, of course! Despite their view of suicide as a symptom of mental illness, Calvin Leeman (2009) quotes a former President of the American Psychiatric Association as saying that many "experts" on dying, including physicians, have either made quiet arrangements with their own doctors or have arranged to have a store of pills available. Suicide is ok for them, but not for us!

Objection 2: Are Those with Psychiatric Disorders Incapable of Rational Thought?

The Role of Insight into the Disorder

There is a well-known joke that you may have heard. A man was driving in the rain along a country road and gets a flat tire. He gets out in order to change the tire, and he notices that he is parked outside a psychiatric hospital, and there are patients strolling around (with umbrellas, of course). Some come to the fence to watch him. He jacks the car up, takes the nuts off the wheel, put them in the hubcap and, as goes to the trunk to get the spare tire, he accidentally kicks the hubcap, and the four nuts disappear into a muddy ditch, lost forever. He is stunned. How can he attach the spare tire to the axle? One of the psychiatric patients says, "Hey Buddy, just take one nut from each of the other three wheels and use those to attach your spare wheel." "That's brilliant," the man said. "I would never have thought of that. But how did you think of it? You're a psychiatric patient here, aren't you?" The patient replied, "I'm here because I'm crazy; not because I'm stupid."

How can I persuade you that psychiatric patients, even schizophrenics (people who have the most severe symptoms such as hallucinations and delusions) can think rationally?

Schizophrenia, a psychosis, often involves a thought disorder and a lack of contact with reality. So what happens if schizophrenics gain some insight into their disorder? Does this insight help the schizophrenics adjust to life and fill them with hope? Apparently not! It had long been observed that insight seems to fill them a sense of resignation and despair which leads to hopelessness and an increased risk of suicide. Some commentators do not necessarily view this as evidence for rationality (e.g., Wilson & Amador, 2007), but it suggests rationality

---

[1] www.oikos.org/mosher.htm.

to me. The lives of schizophrenics can be hellish and, as long as they can remain unaware of their plight, then perhaps their lives are more bearable. But gaining insight into the disorder may be similar to gaining insight into the fact that we have an incurable cancer. Some cancer patients choose to try any and all treatments and "fight" the cancer. Others decided to forego that pain and suffering of the cancer (and the pain and suffering of the treatment), even to the point of choosing to die by suicide. If we consider that decision to be rational, surely the decision of a schizophrenic to avoid the pain and suffering of schizophrenia (and the reduced quality of life) is also rational?

Insight entails three components: (i) awareness of the illness itself, (ii) awareness of the need for treatment, and (iii) awareness of the consequences of the disorder. Components (i) and (iii) are the most likely to lead to hopelessness and despair. Kim and colleagues (2003) studied 333 patients with chronic schizophrenia and asked whether they were aware that they had a mental illness that is due to a biological basis, how hopeless they felt, and their suicidal behavior in the prior month. Recent suicidal behavior was associated with greater hopelessness and more insight into their disorder.[2] Their score on an intelligence test was not associated with whether or not they had engaged in recent suicidal behavior. In a paper I wrote with Maurizio Pompili (Pompili, et al., 2007), we concluded that:

> In summary, research to date suggests that awareness of illness is indeed associated with increased suicide risk in this population, but only if that awareness leads to hopelessness. This conclusion is consistent with the literature demonstrating the relationship between hopelessness and suicide....and helps to reconcile those research findings with the positive prognostic implications of improvement in awareness of the illness.....The severity of the hopelessness that a person with schizophrenia experiences seems contingent, at least in part, on the level of premorbid functioning and the magnitude of the decline in functioning relative to that premorbid capacity. (p. 6)

Therefore, the more aware schizophrenics are of how much the disorder has affected their life and the more severe the impairment, the more hopeless and suicidal they feel.

The vast majority of psychiatrists view suicide as an indicator that a person was mentally ill. Eli Robins (1981) diagnosed almost all the suicides whom he studied after their death, knowing their cause of death, as psychiatrically disturbed. In all the studies in which psychiatrists have diagnosed suicides after their death, they have known the cause of death. No post-mortem study of possible mental illness in suicides and a comparison group (say those who died in single car motor vehicle crashes) has been done in which the psychiatrists did not know the cause of death! Furthermore, some diagnoses, such as borderline personality disorder and the affective disorders have suicidal behavior as one of the cluster of symptoms defining the disorder, which means that an explanation of suicidal behavior using these diagnoses is a circular argument and, therefore, meaningless.

If psychiatrists view the suicides of individuals who have a mental illness as controlled or coerced by the illness, then it is very difficult to explain why only a tiny proportion of those with mental illness die by suicide. Estimates vary for this proportion, with 5% of the deaths of schizophrenics from suicide a commonly cited proportion. I conducted an analysis which showed that, if we were to wait for the whole cohort of schizophrenics to die (rather than

---

[2] And also substance abuse.

working out the proportion of deaths from suicide after a five-year or ten-year follow-up), then the proportion was only 0.5% for male schizophrenics and 0.2% for female schizophrenics (Lester, 2006). Suicide, therefore, is quite rare even in schizophrenics.

Rational thinking in Schizophrenia

Hewitt (2010) pointed out that psychiatrists view schizophrenics (who have the most severe psychiatric disorder) as globally irrational, that is, irrational in every aspect of their thinking and reasoning. As such, they cannot be viewed as having autonomy. Whereas those with medical illnesses can refuse treatment, if psychiatric patients refuse treatment, this is seen as evidence of their irrationality, and treatment can be forced upon them. Is there any evidence that schizophrenics have global irrationality? Hewitt argued that there is none and that schizophrenics can think rationally in many aspects of their life.

In England, there is a law that governs the treatment those with organic diseases of the brain (including intellectual disability [mental retardation] and dementia) called the Mental Capacity Act. Under this act, individuals are judged to lack capacity when they are unable to make decisions because of impairment or disturbance in the functioning of the mind or brain, either permanently or temporarily. They cannot understand or retain relevant information, cannot weigh that information in order to make a decision, and cannot communicate that decision to others. This Act is not applied to mental patients in England, but it would seem a good idea to do so.

One problem with this Act is that there are no agreed upon procedures to assess this capacity. Research, however, has found no evidence that psychiatric patients lack capacity. Cairns and her colleagues (2005) interviewed 112 newly admitted psychiatric patients, and only 44% were judged to lack mental capacity. These patients more often had delusions (but not hallucinations) and more severe symptoms, but less insight. They were more often diagnosed with psychosis and mania. Kemp and colleagues (1997) compared the ability of patients with delusions to normal individuals on tests of logical reasoning. Both groups made errors, and there were no overall differences between the two groups in the number of errors. Owen and his colleagues (2008) examined 338 psychiatric patients using the Mental Capacity Act criteria and found that 40% had the capacity to make informed decisions about the treatment needed. This percentage varied by diagnosis, from 96% for those with a personality disorder to 19% for patients with schizophrenia and 3% for patients in the manic phase of bipolar affective disorder. Finally, Owen and his colleagues (2007) found that schizophrenics performed *better* than healthy individuals on a test of syllogistic reasoning!

Hewitt concluded that psychiatric labeling permits psychiatrists in the UK to force treatment onto psychiatric patients and override the patients' autonomy. This is immoral. It is less of a problem in the United States, since psychiatric hospital beds have been drastically cut over the last few decades, without a comparable increase in community facilities to take care of the psychiatric patients who can no longer be provided with a hospital bed. The net result has been the "lodging" of psychiatric patients in jails and prisons. For example, *The Economist* (August 3, 2013, p. 24) noted that in Cook County (Illinois), the county in which Chicago sits, there are between 2,000 and 2,500 people with diagnosable mental illnesses in the jail.

Mental versus Physical Pain

Hewitt (2013) noted that mental pain is not given equal weight by physicians as physical pain. The medical model, which is a belief system of most psychiatrists, proposes that mental illness have physiological causes, primarily in the brain, and can be cured using psychiatric medications. We could hoist psychiatrists on their own petard. If they believe that mental illnesses have physiological causes, then they are similar to medical illnesses and, therefore, the pain of mental and physical illnesses are both "real."

Hewitt argued that, in order to be rational, suicide must be viewed as an understandable reaction to life circumstances by others; be associated with unendurable suffering; be in accord with a reasonable appraisal of future outcomes in terms of a cost-benefit analysis; have some connection with reduced life expectancy; and be unaccompanied by psychological dysfunction. Others have added that the decision must be free of severe emotional distress. I would argue that the views of the "others" mentioned by Hewitt above are immaterial. We may choose to take into account the views of those others but, for most decisions in life, we are free to disregard their views. I would also argue against the role of psychological dysfunction. Having had cancer myself, which was not terminal, I can assure you that my cognitive functioning was impaired and that I was in severe emotional distress. Severe medical illnesses do not differ greatly from mental illnesses in these respects.

Hewitt noted that the thought disorder and break with reality in schizophrenics (and other psychotic individuals) is not global. Typically, the thought disorder is isolated in a small, discrete domain. For example, schizophrenics with delusions are not delusional about everything or at random. Outside of this discrete domain, schizophrenics can make intentional, reasonable and rational decisions about many issues. Furthermore, symptoms are not always continuous. Individuals with mental illnesses have periods of good functioning and periods of worse functioning.

It is not true that all psychiatric patients can be treated and their symptoms removed. Indeed, psychiatrists write many scholarly articles about "treatment resistant" patients, seemingly blaming the patient rather than themselves for the patients' failure to improve. In addition, psychiatric medications have side-effects which may depress the quality of life. In the 1980s, schizophrenics were given phenothiazines which resulted in the symptoms of Parkinson's Disease. Lithium given to creative individuals with bipolar affective disorder (manic-depressive disease) diminishes their creativity which, for a creative artist, takes the meaning out of their lives.[3] I have friends who were given Prozac and other similar medications (the SSRIs), one of whom drinks a bottle of Pepto-Bismal a day because of the stomach distress, and another who refused to take it because she felt it deadened her mind. Hewitt noted that psychiatrists sometimes use coercion to make patients take their medication, which patients report as dehumanizing and humiliating. Compulsory hospitalization, the use of physical and chemical restraints, and isolation rooms make psychiatric hospitals similar to prisons, as Szasz (1974) has long argued.

Hewitt reminds us that psychiatric patients, especially those with severe disorders, experience "loneliness, daytime inactivity, unemployment, psychological distress, and difficulties with sexual expression. They are and will remain poor and marginal members of

---

[3] Many creative individuals have refused to take the lithium, including the poet Anne Sexton and the yippie Abbie Hoffman, both of whom later died by suicide.

the society until their death. They live in a permanent state of hopelessness and existential distress which is based on a reasonable appraisal of their future prospects. They face stigma from others and the prospect of numerous relapses once they are released as "in remission." Werth (1996) and others have argued that the suffering caused by chronic mental illness may be equivalent to the suffering endured by the terminally ill.

Hewitt does not agree that all those with psychiatric disorders are capable of making rational decisions. She limits those who can make rational decisions to those who are (i) not acting impulsively, (ii) not under extreme emotional distress, (iii) not acting because of delusions or command hallucinations (telling them to jump in front of a train, for example), (iv) capable to make cost-benefit appraisals of alternative courses of action, (v) perceive their situation as unendurable, (vi) have a realistic perception of death, and (vii) do not have conditions that are treatable or remediable.

Objection 3: But Mental Pain is not Real Pain!

This issue was discussed by Hewitt above. Many people, mental health professionals and the general public, view the pain and suffering associated with terminal illnesses as sufficient cause for the decision to die by suicide, but not mental pain. Is this reasonable? As I have argued above, I think not.

Jean Jackson (1992) studied a pain center and found out that those treating them take a multidisciplinary approach involving physical therapy (exercise, ice massages, and transcutaneous nerve stimulation), cognitive therapy (relaxation training and biofeedback), and psychotherapy (individual and group). When she talked to the patients there, she found that many objected to the treatment since it implied that their pain was not real, but in the mind. Physical pain has a mental component too, it appears, a view held by other physicians (Sullivan, 2001).

A Case Study

There is a recent case in which schizophrenics as a group thought and made proposals that were more rational than those of normal people (if one considers those in local government normal).

In June 1997, the Schizophrenia Society of Ontario endeavored to get the Bloor Street Viaduct in Toronto fenced in, to prevent people jumping to their death from it, after they had learned that four of their members had committed suicide from the bridge.[4] This bridge, formerly known as the Prince Edward Viaduct, had been the site for 74 suicides and 16 attempts since 1990.[5] On October 30, 1997, Martin Kruze, a 35-year-old man who went public with his experiences as a teenager of sexual abuse at the hands of employees at the Toronto Maple Leaf Gardens, committed suicide from the bridge. Several suicides followed in the next few weeks, including a 17-year-old student at St. Michael's Choir School.

---

[4] There is also danger from the suicides to cars passing under the bridge.
[5] The figures 37 and 93 have also appeared in newspaper reports. About 300 people have jumped since its construction in 1919. It accounts for half of all bridge suicides in Toronto.

Other strategies proposed for suicide prevention at the Bloor Street Viaduct included emergency telephones distributed across the bridge, police and community patrols, and changing the public perception of the bridge. There are reports of other bridges with telephones: the Mid-Hudson Bridge in Poughkeepsie (NY), the Coronado Bridge in San Diego (CA), the Golden Gate Bridge in San Francisco (CA), the Howard Taft Bridge (DC), the Gateway Bridge in Brisbane (Australia), the Clifton Suspension Bridge, Bristol (UK) and the Erskine Bridge (Scotland). There is a bridge patrol for the Golden Gate Bridge, but no fence.

Different groups lined up on the two sides regarding the construction of a fence. In opposition were the Toronto Historical Board and pro-life groups. Opponents argued that people would simply switch methods if the bridge was fenced in, fencing would deface this landmark bridge, the money involved could be put to better use, and the measure would lead to all bridges being fenced in. In favor were the Toronto Police Department and mental health groups. The Schizophrenia Society solicited letters of support from experts, including Dr. Isaac Sakinofsky at the local Clarke Institute of Psychiatry and myself.

A petition obtained 1,200 signatures, and supporters visited over 46 city councilors in the winter of 1998 to solicit their support. On July 8, 1998, the 57-member city council voted unanimously to hold a design competition for the fence, and $1.5 million was budgeted for the fences and telephones. A luminous veil design from Derek Revington won, and the council approved the design on October 1, 1998.

A subway track runs under the road level of the bridge, and the Toronto Transit Commission objected to the barrier since it would interfere with their inspection of the track which was done by means of a truck with an articulated arm parked on the road level which the fence would have impeded.

The Schizophrenia Society and its supporters worked hard to gather support for the fencing. On March 31, 1999, the Urban Environment and Development Committee approved funds for a modified truck for the Transit Commission. The architects increased their estimates of the cost of the fencing to $2.2 million, and on May 12th, 1999, the Council approved this. Construction of the fence was to have been completed by 2000.

But, then, in the Fall of 1999, the bids for the bridge came in at $5.5 million, and the new Works Committee was composed of city councilors unfamiliar with the project. The Schizophrenia Society once more had to seek support for the project, both in the local community and from experts around the world. The project was once more put on-hold.

The safety fence (called *The Luminous Veil*) was finally funded in 2001 and completed in 2003, after six years of effort by proponents of the fence. As of 2005, there had been no suicides since its construction. Two facts are important here. First, the Luminous Veil received a Canadian national engineering award for design excellence and it is thought to have improved the aesthetics of the Bloor street viaduct.

Second, with regard to cost, John Bateson of the Contra Costa Crisis Center in California has pointed out that cost was not an issue when $5 million was spent to build a barrier to separate cyclists from cars on the Golden Gate Bridge (no cyclists have ever been killed on the bridge), nor when a meridian was installed to prevent head-on collisions (from which there had been only 40 fatalities as compared to 1,300 suicides).

In this case, therefore, schizophrenics displayed more common sense than government officials!

Let us now to run to Martin Manley's essays.

Part 2: Martin's Essays

Chapter 5

Martin's First Entry[1]

My new year's resolution is to explore the idea of committing suicide sooner rather than later - meaning don't just put it off until I become too old to matter to anyone or too old to record my life for posterity.

My first step is to have a discussion between Len Tinman and Al Marley. (Combined anagrams for Martin Allen Manley). Whether this discussion ever sees the light of day, I have no idea at this time. I'm just making sure that if the day ever comes when I end my own life, that this initial and formal thought process is part of the record.

Back in the late 1990's when I first realized that I needed a handle for the internet, I decided that I should use Len Tinman and Al Marley depending upon the site and the reason. Both had their individual personalities. I used Len Tinman when I wanted to have a long-standing relationship and thousands of people know me as Len Tinman. I used Al Marley for more hit and run and confrontational situations. The reason I chose Len Tinman as the "good guy" was because "Len" reminded me of Len Dawson - who along with George Brett and Tom Watson, is arguably the most popular sports personality in Kansas City. In addition, "Tinman" is right out of Wizard of Oz and I live in Kansas.

Len Tinman: Why have you decided now to explore this rather than in the past or waiting until sometime in the future.

Al Marley: Mainly because I haven't had any prevailing reason to do it in the past. As to why not put it off longer, the reason is because the day may come sooner than I would hope when I simply won't be in control of my future.

Len: What do you mean you won't be in control of your future?

Al: I mean someone else will be in control. I'll be too old to make my own decisions. But, that's not the only issue regarding the future. Even if I was in control of pulling a trigger or not, I may have gone beyond my ability to produce a record of my history - proof that I existed.

Len: What difference does it make whether there is a record of your (er... *our*) history?

Al: It makes a big difference to me! Look, I don't have any normal way of leaving a legacy. By that I mean most people have children, lineage. They can live by way of their children's memory as they pass down stories to their own kids. I don't have that.

---

[1] For Martin's essays, I have corrected spelling mistakes, but I have left the punctuation etcetera unchanged.

Len: Ok, so what do you have in mind for a record of your history?

Al: I don't know. I just started thinking about this seriously today.

Len: Let me see if I have this straight. You want to commit suicide because you don't have any children.

Al: That's twisting what I said. First of all, I'm not saying I want to commit suicide – and certainly not today. But, I *AM* saying that I want to begin to consider it seriously. And, the reason is because if I am going to leave a record of my life – whether the world cares or not – I'm going to have to be *proactive* about it. That means I'm going to have to do it while I'm still somewhat lucid, somewhat intelligent. If I wait too long, not only will it be too late to produce it, but it may even be too late to commit the act.

Len: Why is it that you feel you need to leave this documentation of your life when almost nobody else feels that way? Besides, you are saying that you need to do it in lieu of having kids. How can having kids act as a substitute for a documentation of one's life? After all, the kids will eventually die. The grandkids will forget and then the grandparents are lost to history anyway.

Al: Fair question, but I'm not like everybody else. If I was, I'd have kids. And, if I had kids, I wouldn't even be thinking about suicide because there would be too many reasons why I shouldn't. The simple fact is that I believe I have a right to leave a documented history of my life for the world to see or ignore. If I don't, then what was the point of having taken up space on this earth for 58 years?

Len: Most people who believe in the afterlife would say they take up the space on earth for X number of years because that's what God destined. They have a mission during that time and it's not for them to ask "Why?" If they don't believe in the afterlife, they take up space because... they take up space. There doesn't need to be a reason other than simply enjoying life as long as it exists.

Al: Well, as I say, those people aren't me! I *do* believe in the afterlife and I understand God has a destiny or a plan. However, I have to make decisions about a thousand things every single day. What's one more? Besides, I believe if I live to be 70 at the rate I'm going, I will be a babbling, drooling old man in a wheel chair at a nursing home. Not only will I be of no value to anyone, I will be a negative drag on society. Even worse from my perspective, I won't have anything to show for my life by way of documented record and nobody will care and I will be forgotten... forever. Unacceptable!

Len: You are making some pretty broad assumptions. What evidence do you have that you will be that far gone mentally?

Al: The only thing I can say is that nobody alive is more analytical than I am. I know what I can do on a daily basis. I know how many mistakes I make when I type or write or remember or think. I chart everything. I understand trends. I'm making an educated decision that my mind is deteriorating at a rapid rate. I've seen it before with Frank and I'm not going down that road – not a chance in million.

Len: I understand that, but what I do *not* understand is how you can know that this would happen at 60 or 65 or 70 or whenever. Dad was pretty darn sharp at 80! We are a lot like him. Why should we be different?

Al: I'm 100% confident that we're different. He didn't drink two-liters of pop every day for 30 years! Actually, I'm not sure pop ever swallowed a drop of pop. He didn't have a fraction of the astronomical amount of data shoe-horned into his brain that we have had. All I know is that my mind is slipping by the day and if I don't take the bull by the horns and plan ahead… sometime in the not-to-distant future I'm going to wake up one day and I'll no longer be in control and the idea of leaving a documented record of my life will be a hopeless fantasy. And, *THEN* is when I'll be depressed assuming I'm more than a vegetable and even capable of depression. Just as from dust to dust, I'll be going from goo goo ga ga to goo goo ga ga. They'll probably drag my life out for years and years while I have to live with the realization that I'll be just like every other Tom, Dick or Harry that lived on this earth that nobody remembers.

> "In view of the fact that the number of people living too long has risen catastrophically and still continues to rise.... Question: Must we live as long as modern medicine enables us to?... We control our entry into life, it is time we began to control our exit." — Max Frisch

Len: It sounds to me like you've already made this decision, but I've got 50% of the vote.

Al: No, I haven't made the decision. I'm simply saying that it's time to think about it. We don't have any kids. Our parents are deceased. Our brother and sister live in other cities. Neither of them have kids. Most of our friends are analytical enough (or they wouldn't be our friends) that they *might just possibly* understand. Speaking for me, I don't like the idea of using up all our assets and resources for the next 10-20 years when they could go to someone who could use them today.

Len: The problem is that little issue of being born with an innate desire to stay alive as long as humanly possible. You can't simply suppress that by way of some logic.

Al: Oh yes I can! Maybe *you* can't, but that just means you're weaker than me. I'm the left side of the brain and I can easily make the most logical decision irrespective of any emotional issues. It isn't that I don't appreciate the gift of life. I do. It's *incredible*. But, guess what. We're all also given the gift of death. It's *inevitable*. So, why go out with a whimper? Why go out with a bunch of other geezers that nobody knows or remembers? Why not go out with a bang (pun intended)? Why not leave something for the world to chew on?

Len: The reason is simple. Human beings want to live because that's all we know. Every day we want to see, learn or experience something that we hadn't seen, learned or experienced before. If we die, we lose the chance to do that. That's pretty basic.

Al: It's also pretty flawed logic. No matter *when* we die, that will be true. I don't care if we live to be 100, it will be true. It would be true if we lived to be a thousand. There will always be something to learn or experience for the first time. Besides, I don't care about the *quantity* of time I live, I only care about the *quality* of the time I lived… AND I want to make sure I've left a legacy of some kind.

Len: Since I don't know exactly what you are thinking by a record or documentation or legacy for posterity, I'm not sure how to argue that. But, it seems like it could be done two years from now or four years or six years before we were too far gone to be able to write some autobiography.

Al: Maybe so. Maybe no. I'm simply saying I'm going to start thinking about it. Besides the potential problem is that we would wait until we were still barely able to do it, but then we find we can't. I wonder how many millions of people failed to act early enough.

Len: Suppose we decided to pursue this documentation-of-life/ending-of-life scenario, it's going to be hard to get all that done with a full time job and a blog.

Al: Finally, you are making some sense. I agree 100%. It could never work. As you know, we are getting more and more tired all the time. There are only so many hours in a day. We would have to quit the Star – obviously - *way* in advance, but it seems to me we would want to continue with the blog in one form or another right up to the last minute because part of the legacy would the blog. I don't know how we yank Upon Further Review away from the Star, but maybe it could be done.

Len: It sounds to me like you're a hell of a lot farther along with this in your mind than I would have thought. Since I share half your brain…

Al: …what's left of it…

Len: …I'm not quite sure how you have managed to keep me in the dark up to this point.

Al: You are the glass half-full and I'm the glass half-empty. You see what you *want* to see. I see what you *refuse* to see. You think just because we write these complicated sophisticated articles every day on UFR that we're as sharp as ever and as sharp any other 58 year-old. But, I know what it takes. It takes having Google as part of our brain. It takes going over something 10 times that should have only taken once… and 10 years ago *would* have only taken once.

Len: Well, so what? Everyone gets old. Everyone loses their memory. Everyone fades from the front pages of life. It's inescapable and it's part of the cost of doing business as a human being. It seems to me the better way is to accept that fact and go out with dignity.

Al: That's the whole point, going out as a blabbering, slobbering old man in a wheel chair in a nursing home is hardly dignified!

Len: I'm willing to agree to this much. You take a few months and think about this whole thing and I'll do the same. But, the odds of you convincing me to take our life for no other reason but that you think you won't be able to document it at some point in the near future because we are too far gone mentally… the odds of you convincing me of that are slim.

Al: Ok, fine. But, if I can show you over say the next few months (or so) clear and indisputable evidence of our serious mental decline, then I'm going to be a lot more aggressive about this than I even am today. All I'm doing now is simply saying that this issue needs to be looked at closely. I've always been one to be prepared and there is only one chance to be prepared for old age and that's before it's too late to be prepared. I'm not going to just sit idly by and drift with the winds of time into obscurity. No matter what *you* think today, that's *never* going to happen!

My Thoughts

In this witty internal dialogue, Martin addresses the issue of why he is leaving these essays on a website. He has no children, and it seems as if this will be a type of legacy. But for whom? Me and you? It reminds me of an eccentric individual, Arthur Inman (1895-1963), who had a personal crisis of some kind while at college (he never tells exactly what it involved), after which he more or less permanently kept to an apartment in Boston and wrote a diary that he wanted preserved for posterity. He wrote approximately 17 million words, and Daniel Aaron (1985) published a two-volume abbreviated version of the diary. Inman hoped that his diary would be of interest to social historians. Inman killed himself, and his diary does provide some interesting insights into the mind of a suicidal individual (Lester 2010).

Martin says that he would not be thinking about suicide if he had kids. Marsha Linehan and her colleagues (1983) devised a psychological questionnaire to measure, as she called it, *reasons for staying alive when you're thinking of killing yourself*. The questionnaire has subscales to measure survival and coping beliefs, responsibility to family, moral objections, fear of suicide, child-related concerns, and fear of social disapproval (FSD). Martin seems to focus on his responsibility to a family and child-related concerns but, as divorced man with no children, these concerns do not apply.

Martin is showing signs of aging, which seem pretty normal as far as he tells us. We all slow down and forget things more often as we age. Martin, however, is extrapolating these changes to senile dementia in the future. There are no signs of any dementia right now, but what if.......?

His concern raises two interesting questions. What has he experienced in others in his life that makes this such a powerful fear? His father was still intellectually sharp at age 80. But how did his father (and his mother) die? Did they have slow deaths and get dementia? Or maybe his grandparents? Second, he is divorced. So far, we have no idea as to his social support network – does he have one, how big is it, and does he have any really close and intimate confidantes? Maybe he has no one to talk to about these concerns? Married couples typically talk about these issues and plan for the day when they might have to change their living arrangements, such as moving to assisted living and to a nursing home.

I am reminded on a couple I read of when I lived in Buffalo who died by suicide by going over Niagara Falls. They wrote a letter to the local newspaper saying that the husband had terminal cancer and his wife did not want to live without him. By chance, their bodies were found, and the autopsy showed that the husband did not have cancer. It was the fear of cancer that motivated their suicides. In this first entry from Martin, it seems that it is his fear of dementia that is driving him rather than dementia itself.

Chapter 6

I Am Not a Conformist[1]

A little over 20 years ago, I recall there were several things that happened about the same time when I didn't want to do something someone else wanted me to do - and I determined the only reason they wanted me to do it was because it was what everyone else did. I'm sure I had known for a long time prior those episodes that I wasn't like everyone else, but at the time I decided to put it into words to tell others and to remind myself.

I have worked my whole life to figure out who I am, what makes me special, what makes me unique, and how I fit into society as an individual. Having learned who I am, I have become very comfortable and confident of my place. I don't succumb to peer pressure and I won't be intimidated.

There is zero chance that I am going to wake up tomorrow or anytime soon and decide that I am no longer motivated to be different or that I am motivated to being the same as everyone else. I not only don't want to be the same as *everyone* else, I don't want to be the same as *anyone* else! I am not going to do what everyone else does just because they do it. In fact, if anyone else does it, then I am likely to want to do the opposite just to be different.

"Same" follows, "different" leads.

I have succeeded in life to the degree I have because of who I am. I have also failed in life to the degree I have because of who I am. But, one thing is for sure, I am who I am and I'm not anyone else. I live within my own skin and I like it that way.

People remember me because I am different. My tombstone will not read "Here lies another Joe." I don't follow the crowd. I am not a sheep being led to the slaughter. Trends mean nothing to me - unless I set them.

I don't approach things like most others. I am an original thinker. That is why I have accomplished things that others have not. That mindset is what allowed me to invent a few things and to write my books. I am not constrained in my mind by the limits of typical thought and typical behavior. I consider myself to be evolved beyond such a simplistic existence.

I am not going to worry about keeping up with the Joneses. I am not going to care what the Joneses think. I am not on this planet to please the Joneses, but to please myself and

---

[1] This entry is dated June 11, 2012.

whomever I make a commitment to. If a person requires that I become something that I am not, then I cannot make a commitment to them.

So, as a nonconformist, I run the risk of being labeled eccentric, peculiar or even strange. But, many of the greatest personalities and minds in history were off beat... if not off their rocker. That trait is what set them apart from the crowd in the first place and allowed them to reach their full potential - not encumbered by the constraints of society.

> I shall be telling this with a sigh.
> Somewhere ages and ages hence.
> Two roads diverged in a yellow wood and I
> Took the one less traveled by.
> And, that has made all the difference.

Perhaps not surprisingly, that's the only poem I ever learned that I did not write.

My Thoughts

Here, in this brief entry, we get a sense of why Martin is writing these essays about his decision to die by suicide. He is a nonconformist and, perhaps, he hopes that his website will establish (or confirm) the image he has of himself.

Chapter 7

Suicide Preface

I know the question you are asking. "Why did you want to die? ... or Why didn't you want to live?" Here is the answer. I didn't want to die. If I could have waved a magic wand and lived for 200 years, I would have. Unfortunately, that's not an option. Therefore, since death is inevitable, the better question is... do I want to live as long as humanly possible **OR** do I want to control the time and manner and circumstances of my death? That was my choice (and yours). I chose what was most appealing to me.

Let me ask **you** a question. After you die, you can be remembered by a few-line obituary for one day in a newspaper when you're too old to matter to anyone anyway... OR you can be remembered for years by a site such as this. That was my choice and I chose the obvious.

"One lives in the hope of becoming a memory." - Antonio Porchia

I wish there were a different word for "suicide" because that word has become so stigmatized. But, whether I said "suicide" or "taking my life" or "ending my life" or "beginning my death" or whatever... it still amounts to the same thing.

You will rarely get any details for why a person committed suicide, but that won't be the case with me! In fact, this may be the most detailed example of a suicide letter in history - something to be entered into the Guinness Book of Records! My hope is that it is.

I sent personalized suicide letters and emails to many people I know – letters that should have arrived in the morning of August 15th, 2013 – just hours after I did the deed. I also sent boxes with personal mementos to quite a few people in the hope that they will remember me better.

I've planned to end my own life for as long as I remember. I didn't put a date on it, however, until June 11, 2012. I never accepted the (what I would call...) archaic notion that I should simply die at some point – either in a long drawn out miserable death or in an instant for which I was not prepared. That was an insane thought in my orderly world and I knew the only way I could be confident about going out the way I wanted was to do it at a relatively early age.

I was pretty much comfortable living a somewhat abnormal life because I was simply not willing to make the necessary sacrifices in order to have a more normative life. Besides, I always felt that being different was something to be proud of. Although "normal" is a moving target and is nothing like it was 30 years ago, I stayed well in front of the term for most of my life and wouldn't have had it any other way.

Despite what you might think or what the conventional wisdom is regarding suicide, *none of those reasons apply to me.*

1. I had no health issues. I was only sick three times in my adult life that I can remember – and all three were self-induced (accidental). I didn't miss a scheduled day of work in over 25 years. I had no diseases. I never drank. I never took drugs. I never smoked. Thus, I had no physical problems other than occasional acid indigestion – but, that was usually after eating a whole pan of brownies! So, I admit, I did have brownie issue.
2. I had no legal issues. I had never been arrested, much less convicted. I'd never seen a jail from the inside. Other than traffic tickets, I was a model citizen – or at least I pretended to be and nobody could prove otherwise.
3. I had no financial problems. I sold my house which was completely paid for in 1998. The same year I bought $30,000 in 1/10 ounce gold coins and pre 1965 silver coins. Gold was $300/ounce when I bought it and silver was $4/ounce. Gold went up to $1,700 and Silver to $44 making my stash worth over $200,000. And, I had other assets, including a 401K. Besides, everyone who knows me knew I was extremely cheap. I wanted for nothing.
4. I had no loss of anyone close to me that I couldn't bear. My mom and dad died at elderly ages and neither were unexpected. My brother and sister are healthy and active. I never had anyone die who was extremely close to me other than my parents. Other more distant relatives and secondary friends have died, but nobody close.
5. I had plenty of activities in which I participated – including church choir, monthly poker, friends, family, internet, and SportsInReview.com. I did not feel lonely or in any way unappreciated for who I was.
6. I was not depressed. Anyone who says I was is either ignorant or a liar. I stressed out at times – especially in the workplace, because my tendency was to work myself to death. But, I was "retired" for 18 months before I ended my life and I didn't have any stress during that time. In some respects, I feel like I was retired the last 15 years of my life because doing sports statistics could hardly be considered "work". In any event, I can't imagine anyone being more free of stress than I.

So, the major reasons adults commit suicide – health, legal, financial, loss of loved ones, loneliness or depression… none of those issues are relevant to me and, for the most part of my life, have never been.

I decided I wanted to have one of the most organized good-byes in recorded history and I think I will be successful. The key has always been to do it before it becomes impossible to accomplish what I'm doing now – because then it's too late and I would simply be along for the ride to the inevitable cliff. And, that has always been an unacceptable conclusion to my life. *I became convinced that had I waited even another few years, I would* never *have been able to produce this site.*

So, I created MartinManleyLifeAndDeath.com which is prepaid for five years, as is SportsInReview.com. Whether it gets extended beyond that is up to others. Five years is as long as Yahoo would let me pay in advance.

Naturally, I've wondered what people will think about this. Some might consider it gutsy, courageous and preemptive, but I know from my research that most find suicide so reprehensible they will see it as an act of betrayal and cowardice - not to mention premature. It's common to refer to someone battling cancer as "courageous" as opposed to simply following an instinct to stay alive. If trying to stay alive is showing "courage" then the only word for not trying to stay alive would be "cowardice", right?

But, I decided I didn't have the luxury of caring what anyone else thought – which is more or less my recipe in life anyway. Simply put, nobody can control what anyone else thinks and therefore, I decided I was not going to worry about it. Besides, being dead, why would I care? Nevertheless, I strongly believed that if a person seriously wanted to understand who I was and why I did what I did, they will read this site thoroughly… and if they do, they may very well either change their assumptions and opinions or at the minimum, modify them.

Even if I had lived to be a hundred, I would never have been able to say how much I appreciated my friends or family. Had it not been for them, I doubt I would have lived as long as I did. I was even fortunate to have a good relationship with both of my ex-wives. I was thankful for each of these people and for putting up with me despite being too blunt, too obnoxious or too arrogant... too often.

Trust me. I was content up to the last minute. The only thing I was sorry for is that by dying, I may have reminded you of your own mortality – and that seems to be a big problem for everyone else. Sorry. I also realized that some will say I cheated them out of the opportunity to say good-bye to me, but trust me... I knew what you thought and I knew it up to the last minute. You didn't need to say it.

"Death ends a life, not a relationship." — Mitch Albom

Thanks to all of you – Kent, Jeff, Barby, Mark, Chris, Marissa, Charles, Rick, Tom, Todd, Peter, Mike, Donna, Doug, Scott, Teri, Carol, Kipp, Brian, Craig, Jaime, Lloyd, Steve, Jody, Chris, Bob, Jim, and Joe among others.

I practically lived on the internet over the last 15 years and I made a lot of friends. I probably operated better in that environment than in the "real" world. So, I want to thank all my internet friends for reading my stuff and giving me your honest opinions - and with trusting me with your real names.

It's been my honor! Michael, Bob, Glen, Randy, Sam, Dave, Ming, Victor, Cliff, Wade, Bob, Steve, Harry, Aaron, Andy, Burt, Ben, Josh, Dan, David, Mike, Hank, Evan, Eric, Frank, Jonathan, Nick, Phil, Isaac, Ken, Chris, Dan, Kipp, Stan, Mike, Ryan, Neil, Jim, Phil, Steve, Richard, Roger, Ray, Brad, Zach, Michael, Ryan, Andy, Jack, Brent, Tim, John, Jason, Ken, Jeremy, Matt, Clint, Mark, Jimmy, Alan, Erik, Tanner, Lee, Dan, Christopher, Matthew, Vic.

I know I missed some people. Sorry. Whether finance or sports, nearly every internet friend of mine was male - although in a couple cases, the female had a male handle so she could get respect. Too bad that's the way it is, but... So, for two of you, I hope you recognize your "male" name.

You made life a lot easier and if there is anything I might do for you in the afterlife, I will.

"If you have a sister and she dies, do you stop saying you have one? Or are you always a sister, even when the other half of the equation is gone?" — Jodi Picoult

I'm so glad we had this time together
Just to have a laugh, or sing a song.
Seems we just got started and before you know it
Comes the time we have to say, "So long".
-- Carol Burnett

Love, Martin

My Thoughts

I am entering these essays in the order in which Martin listed them at the side of the home page on his website. This essay is called *Suicide Preface*, but actually it is his final suicide note. In it, he tells us that he has already sent personalized suicide notes to friends that will arrive on the day he died (August 15, 2013). In this essay, Martin gives us the reasons for his decision to die by suicide.

He first eliminates all of the common triggers or precipitating events that are thought to motivate suicides – health, legal and financial, problems, loss of a loved-one, loneliness and depression. He says that he wants to control the timing of his death, the manner and the circumstances. In my discussion of the concept of an appropriate death in Chapter 3, I listed as one criterion for an appropriate death as having a role in your own death. This is clearly the case for Martin. In addition, I noted that some points in time can make death at that time appropriate. I have occasionally thought about that in times of threat (in both cases, airplanes that seemed to be in difficulties), and once I decided that it was a bad time to die (I had many unfinished projects) but the second time I decided that it was just the right time, whereupon I had a mild anxiety attack!

Martin also wants to be remembered. Since he had no children, there will be no heirs to remember him, but he hopes that his website will ensure that he will be remembered "for years." It is interesting to note that this book will assist him in this goal. It will preserve his memory for a few more years beyond the website. Martin's need to be remembered is clear from his sending letters and e-mails to many people, as well as gifts.

Martin also wants to be different and to be known as being different. His previous essay asserted that he was not a conformist, and in this suicide note he says, "I always felt that being different was something to be proud of." His death by suicide at this time in his life, and with the documentation of it on his website, has the function of making him unique. He even hopes to become an entry in the *Guinness Book of World Records* for the longest suicide note ever written. Changing, preserving or creating an image of oneself is often present in the motivations of suicides. Indeed, as I write this book, I am also working with a colleague on book on how the act of suicide may be viewed as a performance or dramatic act, in which individuals stage their suicide to create a particular image of themselves. Martin has done just this with his website and with the plans for his suicide.

Chapter 8

Why Suicide?

I feel confident that if you would simply read the first 12 categories to the left side of this website, you would fully understand, and possibly appreciate, the answer to this question. Nevertheless, it's the first question anyone is likely to ask and so here is an attempt at an initial answer.

Keep in mind that I didn't think it was fully possible to answer "Why?" without answering "Why not?" It is because of that that I also included a discussion on "Why Not?", clickable on the left side of this page.

Even so, here is a simplistic answer. The answer is in part… "Because I can." You may think that's trite and that it doesn't answer the question at all, but hear me out.

1. I always thought I might commit suicide someday. When I considered the options of living to be old and all the negatives associated with that alternative, I knew there was no way on earth I was going to allow myself to deal with such an intolerable situation. In order to guarantee that I avoided it, I also knew that I had to commit the act before I was incapacitated and unable to carry it out.

The thought of being in a nursing home, physically or mentally disabled, was the single scariest thing I had ever thought about - at least on this earth. So, in order to make sure that it never happened, I determined that I would have to end things when I was still semi-intelligent and physically able. That's what I mean by saying "Because I can."

> "One said of suicide, 'As long as one has brains one should not blow them out.' And another answered, 'But when one has ceased to have them, too often one cannot.'"—
>
> F.H. Bradley

It's also true that I wanted to leave on top. What does "on top" mean? Of course, it means different things to different people. I'm inclined to think of it in a sports context because I'm such a sports fan – as is evidenced by my other site – SportsInReview.com.

Very few athletes go out on top – or even close. Most play far beyond their peak and even far beyond their relevance. Often times, it's a sad sight to see. I was beyond my peak, but a ways from being irrelevant. Nevertheless, irrelevancy was on the horizon for me as it is most people at my age - me more than average.

The apt analogy is that I've run the race. I already got to the finish line. I didn't croak on the way. I didn't get embarrassed. I didn't break a leg. I sprinted most of the time and sometimes I slowed to a walk to catch my breath. But, I could see the finish line and I liked it!! The last thing on Earth I was going to do when I got there was... keep going. I completed the race because I went over every hurdle that was in my way. Sometimes I fell. But, I got back up and ran that much harder. Perhaps your finish line is a little farther off in the distance than mine. I don't know. I only know I reached *mine* and when I got there the only thing I wanted to do was rest. And, so I shall.

I began seeing the problems that come with aging some time ago. I was sick of leaving the garage door open overnight. I was sick of forgetting to zip up when I put on my pants. I was sick of forgetting the names of my best friends. I was sick of going downstairs and having no idea why. I was sick of watching a movie, going to my account on IMDB to type up a review and realizing I've already seen it and, worse, already written a review! I was sick of having to dig through the trash to find an envelope that was sent to me so I could remember my own address - especially since I lived in the same place for the last nine years!

One of these days, I would have been in choir at church and the rest of them would have started singing the song we had been practicing for three weeks while I would probably have started singing the Star Spangled Banner. And even worse... I would probably have gone all Christina Aguilera on it.

Someday, I would fall down the stairs or slip in the bathtub or get caught walking in a never-ending circle or driving to the store only to end up in Maine. And, nobody would know the difference - at least for a while.

I didn't want to put super glue in my eyes thinking it was eye drops because I suffer from dementia. I didn't want to exist being unable to type on a keyboard because of Parkinson's or drive a car or recognize the people I love. I didn't want to be beaten to death by an intruder or eaten alive by maggots. If you thought I was going to drift through this type of embarrassment and indignity, you were out of your mind even more than me!

And, here's the clincher... it's only going to get worse!

I didn't want to die alone. I didn't want to die of old age. I didn't want to die after years of unproductivity. I didn't want to die having my chin and my butt wiped by someone who might forget which cloth they used for which. I didn't want to die of a stroke or cancer or heart attack or Alzheimer's. I decided I was gettin' out while the gettin' was good and while I could still produce this website! I've been to the penthouse. It may only be a 10-story building, but I refuse to ride the elevator down to the basement! Nope, I'm going out on top. The rest of you can go out whenever you want.

I could overcome most problems I was encountering on August 15, 2013 – especially when I wrote so prodigiously. I could take my time, check, double check, triple check and then hit "send" or "publish". And, even then, I could still edit it. But, the reality is that I struggled a great deal with things that people should not be struggling with at the age of 59... and I was simply not going to sit idly by while that deteriorated until I became a babbling idiot – although some have *already* given me that title.

Of course, there are other reasons.

2. Not all that long ago I started thinking about what I would leave to this world. Since I figured 90% of my energy, creativity, legacy, etc. was already over, the bigger question became not what else I could do while *alive* to be remembered, but rather what I could accomplish by being *dead.*

I know the older I got, the more I would use up my assets and by the time I died – if I live to the age of my dad before his death (83) - I would have very little-to-nothing to leave for others. I know plenty of people that could use the money now and that was a big motivator for me! I had never been left much money, but I could imagine how welcome it would be to get $10,000 (for example) that a person wasn't expecting. That might make a huge difference in the lives of people who don't have a lot - and I was aware of plenty of people I could help.

It's also true that my life insurance was to expire in 2014 and if I live beyond it, I would not be able to afford or justify getting additional insurance. By dying (regardless of by what means) in 2013, I was able to leave that money to people I cared about. For me, money (beyond basic survival) was only of value to make somebody else's life better!

"I spent half my money on gambling, alcohol and wild women. The other half I wasted." -- W.C. Fields

3. If I wasn't already sick of seeing suffering, the past few months before I died was more than enough – too much. First, hurricane Sandy obliterated the NE. Then a crazy gunman killed 26 at an elementary school in Newtown, Conn. Shortly after that a terrorist attacked innocent people at the Boston Marathon. Then there was an explosion at a fertilizer plant in Texas. And then a devastating F5 tornado in Moore, Oklahoma followed by the largest tornado in world history (2.6 miles wide) in nearby El Reno a few days later. These tornadoes killed kids at an elementary school and three storm-chasers among many others. No discrimination. Each one of these events *seriously* broke my heart.

As I say, I was sick of it. It hurt to watch… and I decided I was watching no more.

"On the day of my judgment when I stand before God and he asks me why did I kill one of his true miracles, what am I going to say? I want it to be over and done with. I do. I'm tired. Mostly, I'm tired of people being ugly to each other. I'm tired of all the pain I feel in the world every day. There's too much of it. It's like pieces of glass in my head all the time…" John Coffey, The Green Mile

Unfortunately, it is likely to get worse - a *lot* worse. I honestly believe I would have seen a dirty bomb go off in a big city or a virus sweep the world or a nuke in the hands of terrorists. I honestly believe I might have seen a tsunami wipe out an American coast or a volcano destroy half of Mexico City or Seattle. These things *are* going to happen someday. But, even if they didn't happen in my lifetime had I tried to live as long as I was able, one thing absolutely, positively *would* happen and there is nothing on this earth that can stop it!

4. Economic collapse is inevitable (see U.S Financial to the left). The United States' annual debt and cumulative deficit is *way* beyond the "out of control" label usually associated with it. It's spiraling into oblivion and it will take society with it. Today the deficit is $16.9 trillion dollars with another $125 trillion of unfunded liabilities such as social security, Medicare, prescription drug and federal pensions. It's hopeless.

I felt pretty good about being prepared for economic collapse – the primary reason being all the gold and silver I owned. But, then one day I realized that all the gold and silver and guns and ammo and dried food and toilet paper in the world wouldn't prevent me from seeing the calamity with my own eyes - either ignoring other's plight or succumbing to it. And, that's something I decided I simply was not willing to live through.

I do not advocate anyone take the same way out that I took – especially considering almost everyone has more identifiable reasons to extend their life than I did. But, if you plan to stick around, then you better plan to watch an economic collapse that will be worse than anything you can imagine.

I've listed four major reasons for what I've done. Of course, there are many reasons *not* to do it for most people, but I discuss those in "Why Not?" to the left side of this page.

"Ordinary people seem not to realize that those who really apply themselves in the right way to philosophy are directly, and of their own accord, preparing themselves for dying and death. If this is true, and they have actually been looking forward to death all their lives, it would of course be absurd to be troubled when the thing comes for which they have so long been preparing and looking forward."

Socrates, Phaedo.

My Thoughts

Note that this and the following essays were most likely written days or weeks before his suicide note in the previous chapter.

This essay reveals a little about Martin's motivations, but also raises several issues. Regarding his motives, Martin is anticipating calamities, personal and societal, but the societal calamities will affect him too. Personally, he has observed signs of aging in himself, and he anticipates dementia and dying in in a nursing home with no dignity left. Societally, he foresees financial and natural disasters that will significantly impact him. He seems to have thought a lot about these possibilities, perhaps to the point of what we call *rumination*. Rumination is not always a good thing. It all depends on what you are ruminating about. As an adolescent, I used to ruminate about winning the Nobel Prize in physics, which was uplifting and motivating. To ruminate about the calamities that are on Martin's mind is going to lead to depression, hopelessness and despair. I wonder if Martin had friends with whom he could discuss his worries who might have been able to help him cultivate a *que sera sera* outlook on life – what will be, will be.

You might think that forgetting your address is a severe symptom, but almost all of us in his age range can give you examples of similar "senior moments." I have had to think about my telephone number, zip code and social security number when asked. I have driven off to a destination in the wrong direction, and walked to the wrong classroom at my college. Most of us come to accept that we will have senior moments. They are inevitable.

Martin also gives us two new motives which are of great interest. First, he wants to "go out" on top, that is, die at or near his peak. What came to my mind as I read that is the suicide of Yukio Mishima (1925-1970), a Japanese novelist who died by suicide at the age of 45. He was physically fit and been acclaimed as a great novelist. His writing was no longer as well-received as it had been, and his body was now beginning to show signs of age. Mishima also decided to stage his suicide. He went to an army base to persuade the soldiers to overthrow the government and restore the Emperor of Japan to full power. They refused, and so Mishima committed seppuku, disemboweling himself and having his assistant behead him

Second, Martin says that he has run his race. He has achieved his goals and has no new goals. It is often dangerous to achieve one's goals without establishing new ones. Remember Paul (Bear) Bryant (1913-1983), the football coach at the University of Alabama who died from a heart attack soon after retiring in 1982. My mentor at graduate school, Abraham Maslow (1908-1970), the founder of the field of humanistic psychology, told me just before retiring that he had just finished the last of the papers that he planned to write some thirty years earlier. He died the next year of a heart attack.

A popular current theory of suicide from Thomas Joiner (2005) proposes three elements that are present in suicidal individuals: (i) thwarted belonging, in which important interpersonal relationships have been broken or ended, (ii) perceived burdensomeness in which individuals perceive themselves as a burden or no longer of use to significant others, and (ii) an acquired capability for self-harm in which individuals have to overcome the fear of pain and death. Martin says that he would have little to leave to others if he lived another twenty years. Even his life insurance was scheduled to expire in 2014. We don't know to whom he wants to leave money, but this seems to be important to him, as it is to most people. Hobart Mowrer (1907-1982), former president of the American Psychological Association had a similar concern when he chose suicide three years after his wife had died. Martin sees himself as more useful to others dead than alive.

Chapter 9

Why Not?

Naturally, a normal person would ask… "Suicide – Why?" The fact that I asked "Why not?" establishes from the very beginning the difference in how I viewed life.

Let's face it. Life is the most important issue to all of us. The absence of being alive is either everlasting life or it's forever nothing. Big stuff. We spend our whole lives contemplating what this means. For many of us, we spend our whole lives preparing for the end. But, no matter how much we think about it, few of us stamp a "use by" date on our lives. I did just that 14 months ago. I stamped "Use by August 15, 2013". To be that clinical is what separated me from the masses.

There are, no doubt, many reasons for a person *not* to commit suicide. I felt the most obvious reason is "Why?" That covers a lot of ground, but the main thing it covers is all the people who would never think about it because there is no prevailing terrible problem in their life that might get them to start thinking that way in the first place.

Personally, I didn't believe suicide necessarily must result from a terrible problem, or problems. For me, it was much deeper and much more intellectual than that. The notion was just part [of] my life and had been for many years. It didn't seem like such a strange way of thinking to me even among those that have most areas of their life in perfect working order - depending upon what reasons were keeping them going.

Frankly, I didn't have any major problem that would cause me to do it. I did it for other reasons. I'm sure there are those that suffer terminal illness or financial calamity or loss of loved ones or serious addictions or fear of going to jail for life or just plain depression. And, I acknowledge any of those reasons might spur them toward suicide. But, I believe some of us who do it simply have a dark side that doesn't allow us to appreciate life – or at least *extended* life - in the same way as others.

In a perfect world, I would do a poll of every one of every age. The answers, depending upon the demographics, would be fascinating. The questions would be 1) Why do you want to live one more year? 2) Why do you want to live five more years? 3) Why do you want to live 10 more years? 4) Why do you want to live as long as possible? You should answer those four questions for yourself.

One reason why I was always somewhat of an oddball is the paragraph above. I was *extremely* analytical. I had an insatiable curiosity that could only be satisfied by scientific analysis. Since I couldn't get everyone in the world to answer my four questions, I simply had to speculate.

It seemed to me there are six major reasons people do not seriously consider suicide.

1. The first and foremost reason is "Why?" In other words, "Why would I even contemplate such a thing?" These people have never considered suicide, don't understand it, are probably happy or at least not depressed, fulfilled by work, family, school or some combination. That person is largely foreign to me and so I can't quite identify.

I ask "Why not?" and it seems logical.

Look, I was (and you are) blips! Literally, nothing more than a blip on the radar screen. We appear in the blink of an eye and then we are gone. Perhaps some of us think about our lives in context of the mechanical revolution or the United States of America. If so, our span of years is somewhat more than a blip - it's a percentage. But, just since Christ, my 60 years was insignificant – not only to the world, but to the timeline. If I looked at my life in the context of how long man has been around or will be around, it's a blip. If I looked at it in context of how long the earth has been in existence, it's not even a blip. It's a nanosecond.

"I do not fear death. I had been dead for billions and billions of years before I was born, and had not suffered the slightest inconvenience from it." — Mark Twain

Therefore, what possible difference could it make whether I lived 60 years, 70 years or 80 years? It made zero difference… except to those around me.

2. And, that's probably the second major reason people don't commit suicide – loved ones. For most of us, we are either married or have children or have parents or close brothers and sisters. Most of us have other people that depend upon us either financially or emotionally. I didn't. None of that was relevant to me. My parents have passed on. I loved my brother and sister, but they are both relatively unemotional compared to the average person and they are fully capable of comprehending my decision even if they don't agree – and they probably don't. They are also independent people, married with their own lives and I didn't live in the same town either. And, neither of them had children, so there wasn't even the issue of how nieces or nephews would be affected. They will survive just fine without me.

3. The third most likely reason people want to stay alive is probably related to wanting to see the future. How will my kids develop? How many grandchildren will I have? Will my Cubs ever win the World Series? Will they make a car that goes forever on cold fusion? Is the earth going to come to a screeching halt at some point for this or that reason? Will we discover alien life? "I want to know!"

I understood that. There were a *lot* of those issues for me. After all, I stated that I was extremely curious – not just about the past or present, but also the future. I wanted to know if the Kansas City Royals were ever going to be good and it would have been a blast to be there when they were. I wanted to know if my ex-step daughters had children and what kind of parents they became. I wanted to know how long our poker group stayed together (24 years and counting). I wanted to know what kinds of technologies were going to make life more interesting or convenient. I wanted to know a thousand things that will happen in the future…

…but that's not enough reason. And, again I point to the blip argument. There will *always* be reasons to want to stay alive another year or five years or 10 years. It wouldn't have mattered how long I lived, there would have been hundreds or thousands of itches to scratch!

Don't think there weren't times every single day when my mind would be tempted to say "I can't wait until (pick a date) to see what happens with (pick a subject)" regarding the future beyond August 15, 2013... but I never wavered for a single second because I always knew that whatever day I died – whether 2013 or 2023 or 2033, I would never have been able to satisfy those thoughts.

4. If I had to have guessed, I would have said the fourth most prevailing reason to stay alive is because of accomplishments. People want to accomplish as much as they can in their lives and they don't want to run out of time before they do it. Of course, for people who think that way, they never fulfill all those accomplishments anyway and they never will. So, the only thing to do is keep chasing them until you die. Unfortunately, the older you get, the less likely you will accomplish existing goals. It's like the guy who retires the day after he wins baseball's triple crown and then the World Series. He goes out on top because he can never be as good again and he can never *feel* as good again. That's how I felt right up to the end. Not that I had done all that much, but one thing is for sure. I would never have been able to do anything greater than what I had done up to that point – unless it ends up being related to this website.

5. The fifth reason is the recently popular term "bucket list" – meaning the things you want to have experienced before you kick the bucket. I omitted "accomplishments" (#4 above) from this list. Bucket list items are things like going on a Mediterranean cruise, touring the White House, fishing for salmon in Alaska, climbing Pike's Peak and on and on and on. Nearly every one of these things require traveling somewhere. Otherwise, they are probably "accomplishments".

I didn't have such a thing. I once had a quasi-bucket list when I was about 22 – things to accomplish by the time I was 30. When 30 came around and I hadn't accomplished them, I decided the bucket list idea was stupid.

For me, a bucket list was a totally arbitrary and manufactured reason to want to stay alive. I'd been to Disney World. I'd skied the mountains in the winter and biked them in the summer. I'd had fun on the Vegas Strip numerous times. I'd swum in two oceans and the Gulf. Big deal. Been there, done that. The list of what I *could* do – like attend the Talladega 500 or the Tour de France – is a mile long. No matter how many things I did, there would still be more on the list. I doubt if anyone alive, who bothers to create a "bucket list", completes it. So, does it really matter if you check off one item or ten items or 100 items when there will always be more on the list? It's like a leaky boat. For every bail of water you toss out, a bail and a half leaks in. When you kick the bucket, your bucket list will die with you – whether it's a quarter full, half full or fuller than full.

6. The last major reason I thought of for why people want to live indefinitely is the whole notion of leaving a legacy. By the time someone is 60 years old, they either have a legacy or have not. There isn't a lot of new opportunities to make a mark by the time you reach that age - Colonel Sanders notwithstanding. I accomplished a few things, left a few legacies. I was mostly satisfied.

Suicides and/or suicide attempts are often (as they say) a cry for help, or a way to punish people they are upset with, or a means of controlling a situation. But, none of that was a reason for me either except that controlling my death was paramount.

So, although most people don't even consider suicide unless there is something terribly wrong, I believed if those same people were forced to give reasons why not, it would be about family and friends that depend upon them, seeing the future, more things yet to be accomplished or experienced and leaving a legacy.

I understood all those reasons and if they had applied to me, I would have been gung-ho for living longer. But, the fact is they didn't apply to me at all. Everyone I knew had some (or all) of these reasons to live. I was happy for them. I truly was. In many ways I learned how to live vicariously through others – not because I wasn't content, but because I always admired anyone that understood how to be truly happy.

> "There are only four things in life that matter. The first is happiness and I'll sell you the other three for a dollar." – Sam Walton

I also always recognized – perhaps more than the average person – how important happiness is. I just was never able to find it for more than brief periods in my life and so I almost never used the word "happy"... I guess because I identified it as an emotion. Instead I found myself using the word "satisfied" which is more of statement of fact – something that can be measured or quantified... like X=4 "satisfies" the equation of $2 + 2 = X$.

Don't misunderstand. I wasn't miserable to the point of depression, but I've never known how to smell the roses the way many other people can. Besides, I really have had everything I could realistically want considering what I was willing to sacrifice in return - way more than I've *needed*. And so, being content with a minimal number of things was very easy for me.

At some point, the issue is less about "more" than it is about not having "less". Michael Jordan has talked about the "joy" of his first championship, but by the third championship, it had become more "relief". Happiness had become the absence of misery – the misery of losing. And, so for me.....

> "Happiness is the absence of misery." – Martin Manley

My Thoughts

Martin tells us that he made the decision to die on his 60th birthday, some 14 months beforehand, and so, clearly, his decision was not an impulsive one. He notes that this separates him from the masses, and this emphasizes Martin's need to view himself as special, which some psychologists would see as a symptom of narcissism. He's a nonconformist and not one of the masses!

And yet at the same time, he is a blip in this world. This is a dilemma for many of us – the fact that we see ourselves as unique (and special), and yet we are one of seven billion individuals currently, let alone all of those who have in the past and who will exist in the future. The experience of being "me" is a subjective experience, while the idea that we are mere blips is an intellectual thought. It is not often that intellectual thoughts become driving forces for our actions. Those who have strong political or religious views sometimes fashion their lives around these views, but they tend to feel passion (and other emotions) about these views. The notion that we are blips does not arouse much emotion, except that Martin talks of having a dark side. Maybe he will tell us more about this dark side later, but he says in this essay that he is not depressed, just generally miserable. He has never found happiness, only occasional feelings of satisfaction. He has had everything he ever wanted, but could never stop and smell the roses.

Although he talks of having friends (and listed many in Chapter 7 above), his parents are deceased and his brother and sister childless and emotionally distant. He does not have strong family ties.

He lists his reasons for not staying alive as: (i) intellectually, each of us is a blip – nothing special, (ii) he has no strong family ties, (iii) he does not care too much about seeing the future, (iv) he has accomplished what can and does not have anything more to accomplish, (v) he has no bucket list of things to do before he dies, and (vi) any legacy he can leave has already been left.

In the end he comes back to what is important for him – controlling his death.

Chapter 10

Why Age 60?

Clearly, age 60 is somewhat of an arbitrary age to end my life. But, it isn't just that age 60 is a nice round number. It's also August 15, 2013 – the very *day* I turned 60. That's symmetry and I loved a lot of things, but not many more than good symmetry.

Besides, beginning with the age of 60, a lot of people begin to die. It's too bad, I guess. I suppose we should all be so fortunate to live to be Methuselah's age of 969, but much like the buggy whip, the glory days of 900+ year olds is a thing of the past.

Famous people who have died younger than 60...

Jimi Hendrix 27, Princess Di 36, Michael Jackson 50, Abraham Lincoln 56, John Kennedy 46, Dr. Martin Luther King Jr. 39, John Lennon 40, Kurt Cobain 27, John Kennedy Jr. 38, Robert Kennedy 42, Elvis Presley 42, Janis Joplin, 27, Thurman Munson 32, Lou Gehrig 37, Heath Ledger 28, Anna Nicole Smith 39, Marilyn Monroe 36, John Denver 53, George Reeves 45, John Belushi 33, Chris Farley 33, River Phoenix 23, Bob Marley 36, Linda McCartney 56, George Harrison 58, Judy Garland 47, Jim Morrison 27, Amy Winehouse 27, Steve Jobs 56, Natalie Wood 43, Freddie Prinze 22, Whitney Houston 48, Steve Irwin 44, Tupac Shakur 25, Bernie Mac 50, Bruce Lee 32, Roberto Clemente 38, Elvis Presley 42, Freddy Mercury 45, Andy Kaufman 35, Patrick Swayze 57, Jesus 32, Babe Ruth 53, Marvin Gaye 45, Buddy Holly 22, Michael Landon 57, Hugo Chavez 58, Andy Warhol 58, James Dean 24, John Candy 43, Jim Croce 30...

...just to name a few. There is no shame in dying at 60.

Even though not being on the government dole is of zero consequence to the future economic collapse of the United States, I could take pride in the fact that I wasn't going to be sucking on the nipple of the federal debt by taking social security and Medicare. When the US economy collapses, it won't have been me that contributed to taking it down.

Besides, if you create a ledger with all the contributions that I would have made to friends, family and society from age 60 on... and you also note all the contributions that friends, family and society would have made to *me* from the age of 60 on, I felt there was a real strong possibility that I would have ended in a net negative - and perhaps much sooner than I would have even expected. By giving everything I have up to the last minute, I knew in my heart that I contributed the most I could possibly give and taken the least I could possibly need.

Another reason why age 60 is ideal is that my life insurance expires next year and I would not be able to afford to get new insurance without paying a ton. And, it requires two years of waiting - once you get insurance - before you can commit suicide and still have the beneficiaries receive the death benefit.

After I got my second divorce, I chose to lease a three bedroom, two bath duplex. It was probably a lot more space than I needed, but at the same time, it was great to have the room. When I first moved in, my lease began September 1st, 2004.

I renewed it every year since. I guess it was just luck instead of destiny, but my birthday was August 15th. That was a perfect day to die - two weeks before my lease expired. Although I planned to have the vast majority of my personal property gone by the time I died, there were a few things for my sister to take care of. I informed my landlord in late July that I would not be extending the lease. That gave my sister two weeks to take the few things I left for her before the lease expired and it gave him time to have it ready to re-lease by September 1st.

And, if that wasn't enough coincidence, my renter's insurance renews on August 31st as does my car insurance as does my driver's license as does the license plate on my car! What are the odds? I always loved it when a plan would come together.

I know it may seem superficial, but I hated winter so bad that to die during a cold, dark icy snow-stormy night would have been the worst possible way to go out. If nothing else, the symbolism sucks! As it is, I got to see another spring and another longest day of the year. By August 15th, I was as far away from winter as it is possible to get. Thank God!

And, finally this. From Star Trek: The Next Generation (Half a Life), 1991. Proof that I was 200 years ahead of my time! From en.memory-alpha.org

David Ogden Stiers (Dr. Timicin) falls for the mother (Lwaxana) of one of the crew on the Enterprise. At first he tries to discourage her from being interested in him, but eventually neither can resist the urge. Unfortunately, their relationship can never last.

Lwaxana becomes livid with protest when she discovers that, approaching the age of 60, Timicin is, upon returning to his planet, to undergo the "Resolution", ritual suicide. She immediately goes to Captain Picard and demands he intervene to spare Timicin's life, but Picard refuses to do so, as he is bound by the Prime Directive not to interfere.

Lwaxana and Timicin spend a lot of time together, discussing the concept of ritual suicide back and forth. Lwaxana considers the practice barbaric, while Timicin attempts to explain that in his culture it is an accepted practice for all to undergo the ritual on their 60th birthday to avoid old age, infirmity, indignity, dependence on others, and the cruel uncertainty about when the end would come.

Each ends up finding the other's point of view cruel: Lwaxana because she sees it as arbitrary murder in an uncertain universe when death can come both well *before* and well *after* the designated age, Timicin because she is denying people control of their fate and the opportunity to end life with dignity.

Despite going back and forth on the issue, Lwaxana eventually concedes, though she still disagrees with the tradition. She packs her bags and sets out to accompany Timicin to the planet to be with him at his ritual. She promises not to cause trouble and Timicin and Lwaxana beam down hand in hand to the planet.

COOL FACTOID: David Ogden Stiers was approaching 60 years of age in real life when this episode aired.

My Thoughts

Again we read of Martin's dread of being a burden, not on any particular individual, a more common concern, but a burden on society by using resources such as social security and Medicare. It is of interest here that most of those whose goal is to prevent suicide talk of the cost of suicide to society in terms of lost wages and productivity. In an article by my wife and me (Yang & Lester, 2007), we worked out that the 32,000 suicides in the year 2005 saved the nation about $5 billion. We didn't argue that we should not prevent suicide. We argued that this should be done on humanitarian grounds and not on economic grounds. We got the idea for our study from a paper by Viscusi (1984) who showed that each pack of cigarettes sold saved the nation about 72 cents because smokers died early, meaning less medical care and nursing home costs and less money received from the government (in the form of social security, etc.).

Martin also likes the idea of dying on his birthday. In studies of the timing of suicide, researchers have noted a *birthday blues* effect. By using the terms *blues*, researchers imply that these individuals are depressed on their birthday, but there is no evidence for that and so the term is a poor choice. However, do individuals tend to die by suicide more than we would expect by chance on or near their birthdays? I reviewed research on suicide up until 1997, and all of the dozen or so studies on this found no birthday blues effect. Nonetheless, for Martin, all of the time-related features, such as renewing leases and licenses, made his 60th birthday an ideal time for him.

Incidentally, Martin is correct about life insurance. Many believe that dying by suicide invalidates your life insurance. It does not. There is usually a two-year period after taking out life insurance during which you do lose benefits if you die by suicide but, after two years, life insurance policies are usually honored by insurance companies.

Chapter 11

Self-Serving?

I wanted to address something that simply *has* to be going through your mind as you look at this site. At least on the surface, I'm sure many readers will consider this to be self-absorbed, narcissistic or even egotism run amok.

Maybe, but here is what you are overlooking – and this is critical. This is to be the *LAST AND ONLY CHANCE* I will ever have to tell the world who I was. I would never have another opportunity to add to my story – not in a year, not in a thousand years.

You may live 10, 20 or 50 more years. You will have plenty of opportunities to make a mark and to leave a legacy. My legacy is over. If I were to simply stick a gun in my mouth and leave nothing to be seen, whatever legacy I had would have evaporated into nothingness in a very short period of time.

"No one is actually dead until the ripples they cause in the world die away..." — Terry Pratchett

Since my entire life of 60 years is on this website along with *SportsInReview.com*, I didn't think there was any reason why I should have felt ashamed of producing this material. If nothing else, think of it as an autobiography – and maybe the first of its kind, but hopefully not the last.

When I was in Florida in 2004 for two months, I got an idea being around all those old people. I thought about how they were going to die off and nobody would really remember them. And, the reason why is because they didn't leave anything tangible about themselves to be remembered by. Not everyone is rich enough or famous enough to leave behind a building or a street with their name on it. Only a very few have a Wikipedia page.

I thought it might be an interesting business to do the kind of work for people that I've done on this site – before they are either too incapacitated to provide the information needed or before they die – whichever comes first. Old people with money seemed like a good opportunity for a business such as this because what's left after a certain point in life besides just playing it out to the end? One thing that *should* be left is to make sure that whatever legacy one has is remembered – that whatever mark one makes is not forgotten.

Naturally, when I thought about this for others, I thought about it for myself. Since I did not have children, I did not have that legacy to leave – something that most people have. And, although it may well be true that the world didn't need a bunch of little Martin Manleys running around, it also meant I couldn't just fade into dust knowing my children would carry on some form of who I was, not to mention keeping my memory alive.

Frankly, the thought that my memory or legacy would come to an abrupt end was unacceptable to me – and in my opinion, it *should* be unacceptable to anyone in my situation.

> "There are three deaths. The first is when the body ceases to function. The second is when the body is consigned to the grave. The third is that moment, sometime in the future, when your name is spoken for the last time." — David Eagleman

I also thought that a clearing house should exist for all the "First Name Last Name Life And Death" sites such as this. It could be called something like Eulopedia.com. That domain name is still available as of August 15, 2013. If you want to read about someone's life with this level of personal detail – no matter how famous they were, simply go to Eulopedia.com, look up the name and go to their "Name Life And Death" site.

It's incredible what is lost to history. Even one generation back, so little is really known about the vast, vast majority of people. It's a shame - especially considering existing technology has enabled us to store everything ever said, done or thought by every person on earth a thousand times over. There is no reason lives have to continue to be forever forgotten. Everyone can be remembered if they put in the effort to be remembered in some concrete form rather than simply being dependent upon fading memories of those who knew the deceased person.

I never claimed to have more to say about myself than millions of other people, it's just that they either aren't thinking about the end game or don't care how they are remembered. And, of course, the reality is that I was highly motivated to do what I did because I started the clock on June 11, 2012 and... the clock was ticking – and really loud. Most people don't hear the clock until it's too late to produce something like this. And, that's been one of the great rewards for planning my death 14 months in advance!

> "The funny thing about facing imminent death is that it really snaps everything else into perspective." — James Patterson

People write autobiographies all the time. Most are, of course, about someone famous. That's the only way it could work up to this point. It takes a lot of time by some second party to work with them as well as the cost to produce it in paper form. To be justified financially, it must have a famous name attached. But, the cost to do *this* site was insignificant – even pre-paying for years in advance. The time *is* extensive, but I had it, so I used it.

The point of this is that with only a brother and sister, no children, no nieces or nephews, I will have been forgotten pretty fast unless I did something that was *way* outside the box. And, so would my parents have been forgotten. At least on this site, I also remembered them. As long as MartinManleyLifeAndDeath.com exists, so do their memories.

And, for that, I do not apologize.

I wanna leave my footprints on the sands of time
Know there was something that, and something that I left behind
When I leave this world, I'll leave no regrets

Leave something to remember, so they won't forget
I was here...
I lived, I loved
I was here...
I did, I've done, everything that I wanted
And it was more than I thought it would be
I will leave my mark so everyone will know
I was here...
Beyonce

My Thoughts

Well, yes, it is somewhat narcissistic. But today, with *Facebook* and *Twitter* and everyone striving for their five minutes of fame, haven't we all become a little narcissistic? Part of the motivation for having children is to carry on one's name and genes and to be remembered by one's descendants. That is narcissistic. I write books and articles that I hope will be read in the future – narcissism. And I will probably renew my website before I die (www.drdavidlester.net). So Martin is in good company.

Martin quotes David Eagleman on three types of deaths. Neat, but not as neat as the four types defined by Richard Kalish in Chapter 3 of this book: biological, psychological, social and anthropological deaths. But if the world ends in a cataclysm for the human race (which is bound to happen within a billion or so years), the records (and memories) of all of us will disappear.

Chapter 12

Suicide – How To

I didn't want to get too gruesome with this, but at the same time if you don't want to read all about it, I suggest going on to the next category! The simple fact is that, despite the bazillion things I had to think through over the last 14 months, the one that ultimately mattered the most was *how to* commit suicide.

Just as I have done regarding many other aspects of this, I researched the subject. I discovered organizations which exist solely for the purpose of helping people do the deed - so to speak. I also found a number of sites that actually rated each way to do it. That was, of course, right up (or is it "down"?) my alley.

I evaluated the pros and cons of all the methods. Fortunately, or *un*fortunately, depending upon your viewpoint, the government makes it hard to get the drugs that would be ideal.

Obviously, many things will kill a human, however many of them take inconsistent amounts of time to "work" and some of them are unpredictable in the results. In fact, some of them might only leave you in a vegetative state. Clearly, that's unacceptable.

Of course, some methods will be so painful, you will wish you were dead. Oh, wait, that's the *goal*. Okay… "you will wish you had never been born."

Nobody wants to suffer during the process – at least I didn't. Hanging sucks. Jumping out of a window sucks. Drowning and burning and freezing are even worse. There are 50 ways to die, but very few which are painless, quick and certain.

One of the ways I thought would be as good as any other was to simply take a bottle of sleeping pills (which I had) and then go sit in the car in the garage, start the engine, and go to sleep. And, that might have been the best option if it weren't for the fact that I had half a duplex. It's very possible the fumes could escape into *their* living quarters and harm or kill them. So, instead of *suicide* as my last execution, it's *murder*! Unacceptable.

Probably the best drug to take would be Nembutal, which I believed could be purchased in Mexico. The problem was the risk that it would be either watered down or fake. The bigger problem is that you won't know if it is "good" until you take it. What if it doesn't kill you?

In my case, I had everything worked out exactly as I wanted it based upon the calendar. I couldn't take any chances that something would go wrong. Suppose I sent out a couple dozen personalized letters via Fed Ex overnight on August 14th and then I screw up. "False Alarm... Just Kidding!" That doesn't cut it in my orderly world!

When push came to shove, there really was only one way to go and that was via a firearm. It's about as certain to work as you can get. Nobody else needs to be involved. It's immediate, it's painless and you can control where you do it.

Of course, even that wasn't as simple as it might seem – at least not to me. I owned two 22-gauge pistols, but both had mechanical problems. Even if they worked, would a 22 kill me? Very possibly not. So, that meant a higher caliber pistol. I was about to go out and buy one, but coincidentally, one fell into my lap about six weeks before I needed it. I took it out and practiced to make sure I had it figured out... the rest is history.

It's one thing to plan all of this and to create this site and all the other things I've done, but when you actually obtain a gun specifically for that reason, it makes what up to that point was theoretical, into something far more concrete. Even though every single day for 14 months I asked myself whether I was sure I wanted to do it and every single day I said categorically "yes", it's still another step to go obtain the pistol that will end my life and even more surreal to pull the trigger knowing the only reason I'm doing it is to make sure I know how to do it one time a few weeks later... a bullet with my name on it.

One of the problems with shooting oneself is the obvious mess. I thought about that a lot. I didn't want anyone I knew discovering my body and I didn't want to make a mess in the house – something my sister or my landlord would have to deal with. No way.

I also didn't want anyone discovering my body or witnessing it who wasn't trained for such a thing. I finally decided the best way to do it would be at 5AM on August 15, 2013 at the far southeast end of the parking lot at the Overland Park Police Station. If everything worked out right – and I'm sure it did, I called 911 at 5AM. I told them "I want to report a suicide at the south end of the parking lot of the Overland Park Police Station at 123rd and Metcalf. Bang."

They should find me in about two minutes. I doubt they will be able to identify me for a couple hours at least which will give my sister time to learn about it before the police would have been able to contact her. There will be a note lying next to me which says:

> I committed suicide of my own free will. I am not under the influence of any drugs. I am sorry for your inconvenience! You will be contacted within a matter of hours by my sister. She will find out about this by an overnight letter and/or email I sent to her which she will get this morning. In it, I explain the exact location where I shot myself and gave her your phone number. At that time, she will tell you who I am. If you discover who I am prior to her call, please do not contact her. I do not want her (or anyone else I sent letters to overnight) to find out about it from *you*. I want them to find out about it from *me*. Thank you!

> In addition, I recently went through a process of donating an organ. Unfortunately, that process could not be completed by this date. PLEASE contact the following people (especially Marilee Clites - the first person on the list) so that they may be able to harvest any organs of mine immediately.

Marilee Clites: Kansas University Medical Center
mclites@kumc.edu, 316-322-5139, 913-945-7755, 816-829-8200
JoAnn Oxman: Kansas University Medical Center
joxman@kumc.edu, 913-558-0266

Melissa Ott: Midwest Transplant Network
 mott@mwtn.org, 913-302-7949, 913-261-6164
Catherine Nash: Midwest Transplant Network
cnash@mwtn.org, 816-519-0216, 913-261-6170

I have sent them emails telling them of my death and begging them to actively try to harvest my organs to save another person(s) life. Please cooperate with them if they call. Thank you!

Also, please destroy this gun, ammunition and phone. They serve no further purpose.

And, finally, I've prepaid for my cremation from D.W. Newcomer's, 8201 Metcalf Ave., Overland Park, Ks. 66204 (913-648-6224). The contact is Roger Breckenridge.

If you are trying to imagine what it was like in the closing minutes - standing there next to a tree in the dark at the corner of a parking lot all by myself with a gun and a bullet... you are worrying too much about what must have been going through my head - no pun intended. I *guarantee* you from having imagined my way through it a hundred times, the only thing going through my head was asking forgiveness, remembering those whom I love, being glad I was able to end it the way I wanted and thrilled to death that I left this website. Don't weep for me dying alone. We ALL die alone.

In my letter to Barbie I explained where the car is parked as well as how to get into my house and many other things. I sent overnight letters and emails to her home and her work so as to be sure I covered all the bases.

The GPS coordinates for the location are: 38 54.135', -94 40.433'.

"Suicide is the role you write for yourself. You inhabit it and you enact it. All carefully staged -- where they will find you and how they will find you. But one performance only." — Philip Roth.

This is the only method and methodology that would work from my perspective. I prepaid for cremation, however I suspected they would do an autopsy on me to make sure I wasn't on drugs. As to what Barbie chose to do after that, it was up to her. All I could do is make suggestions which I did.

The act of suicide can be horrible for those left behind. I couldn't control the fact of the matter, but I *could* control the circumstances. I believe the way I did it, coupled with the overnight letters/emails and this web site, is the best I can do to mitigate the hurt. And, besides, as I said in other categories on this site, if I was seriously needed by anyone or if I had parents or children, I would never have considered it. As it turns out, my daily freedom from responsibilities gave me the *ultimate* freedom.

My Thoughts

Much of my research has been on the choice of method for suicide, and I am currently working on a book with a colleague on how people stage their suicidal act. Martin has given a lot of thought to these issues. He chose a firearm, the most popular method for men in the United States. It is the most lethal method available. It does leave a mess, and I usually hypothesize that, if someone uses by firearm at home so that a significant other will find the body, then the suicidal person is angry at the significant other and wants them to suffer. Martin has considered this issue, wanting to spare his sister and his landlord. And he even gives me a quote from Philip Roth to support the thesis of my book in progress.

The other noteworthy aspect is that Martin has backed himself into a corner. He has sent the suicide notes to friends and an overnight letter to his sister. He plans to call the police and fire the gun while on the line. Once he calls, he has further backed himself into that corner.

Finally, he reiterates how no one needs him. He is free to choose suicide with no reason to stay alive.

Chapter 13

Growing Up

As a child I grew up poor along with my mom, dad, brother and sister. We didn't have much and it would be disingenuous to say we at least had each other. I suppose that's technically true, but I'm not sure how much value there was in having each other - since all that meant was that we shared the same roof.

My mother Bertha was born August 28, 1926. She was 15 years younger than her next youngest sibling. She was, for lack of a better word, an accident. In those days, accidents happened and they didn't get *un*happened, if you know what I mean. Thus, she was mostly raised as an only-child. My father (November 23, 1923) *was* an only-child and he was adopted. Neither of my parents grew up with brothers or sisters. Both lived in an abnormal and somewhat isolated environment for people of their era.

The two began communicating while my dad was stationed in the Pacific during World War II. When he came home, they married. That was June 3, 1946. My sister (Barbie) was born in 1951, followed by myself on August 15, 1953 and my brother (Mike) in 1955. Each of us was born two years and two months apart.

In the 1950's, almost everyone came from a "normal" family environment – meaning two parents and several siblings. However, my mom and dad were both from an *unusual* environment – one where they didn't experience the typical "family" atmosphere.

Consequently, when they had three children, they simply didn't know how to impart the "family" mindset because they hadn't grown up with it. Even so, it's possible we were relatively typical – at least until I was 11. I frankly can't remember that far back. In the summer of my 12th birthday, we moved from a neighborhood in Topeka, Kansas – a neighborhood of hundreds of baby boomers and just a block from the grade school - to a house in western Kansas that wasn't even in a town, but rather nine miles from a small oil spot on Highway 56 called Pawnee Rock where we went to school.

It was culture shock on the highest order. For a young boy just beginning puberty, it was extremely difficult. Before we moved, I could have barely told you the difference between a horse and a cow. Instead of kids my age next door and two doors down and three doors down as far as the eye could see, I had my brother, my sister and sound of moos.

Barbie turned 14 just after we moved and began getting to know kids in the small town where we would be going to school that fall. Girls mature sooner anyway. Add 2+ years of age and the fact that the guys liked her… and you can see I wasn't able to identify with her situation. Not only that, she was learning to drive. Instead I was stuck in the sticks with my younger brother.

My parents both worked. Even worse, my mom worked nights. So, we simply didn't have a normal family time together. Despite my mom working multiple jobs and my dad working, we were always poor. I used to quip that my two favorite toys when growing up were a stick and a rock. And, I would get one sock for my birthday in August and the matching sock for Christmas. We lived in an old farm house and the floor in my bedroom was so sloped that I raced checkers from one end of the room to the other... and kept stats on it!

Due to the environment, I quickly learned how to entertain myself and it eventually culminated in me being extremely self-focused as well as self-sufficient. There was only one thing to do every day – satisfy whatever curiosity I had. In some respects, that became an obsession.

I've always been very mathematically inclined. I love statistics and have spent my whole life dealing with them in one way or the other – if not for my vocation, than for my hobby. I spent thousands of hours as a teenager making up pretend baseball, football and basketball leagues, drawing plays from cut-out pieces of paper in a shoe box and keeping stats for make-believe players and teams.

Even as I got older, I always took the bus home and so I really never spent a lot of time with the kids in town. I can't say I cared. They were a bunch of hicks as far as I was concerned, but then I'm not sure I even knew what a *hick* was – just that whatever Martin Manley was… he wasn't one of them! Of course, I'm sure from their perspective, they were just as happy not to be one of me.

I kept stats for the basketball and football teams at Pawnee Rock high school during my freshman-junior years. I remember being fascinated with our teams and my whole world revolved around how good they were.

During my freshman year, the football team went 7-0 in eight-man football. Every win was by a margin of 40 or more points. There were no high school football playoffs in those days. They came a few years later. But, according to some high school poll somewhere, Pawnee Rock ended the season ranked #2 in the state behind a team that hadn't lost in six years.

That same year, the basketball team was also good, but had lost three times during the season. In the regional finals, Pawnee Rock was behind by 15 points early in the second half – a seemingly insurmountable deficit. However, the team won on a last second shot to go to the state tournament. In the first game at state, Pawnee Rock trailed 21-2 at the end of the first quarter. Early in the second quarter the team was behind 25-2... Oh, the humanity! By halftime, we had cut the deficit to 11. By the end of the third quarter, the deficit was eight. Pawnee Rock eventually took the game to overtime and won! The fact that PR lost the semifinal and third-place games meant very little. If I hadn't been hooked on sports and sports statistics before my freshman year of high school, I certainly was by then.

From the time we moved to western Kansas, we attended a small church in Pawnee Rock. The reason was because one of my father's co-workers in Great Bend was a part-time pastor at the church. My dad was a social worker for the county as was the pastor of this church. His son is Charles and we became life-long friends - a friendship which existed to the day I died.

I went to 7th, 8th, 9th, 10th and 11th grades in Pawnee Rock – a town of about 450 people. My senior year, I transferred to Great Bend (18,000). Instead of being bussed nine miles to school and back, I drove my own car 13 miles.

As a senior at Great Bend, I was able to exist in the background without too much trouble. The downside is that I knew almost no one. There were a few others that had transferred from Pawnee Rock to Great Bend during those years and I knew a few of them. But, again, I really didn't have a group of friends that I felt comfortable with.

I was in the Madrigal-Pops Choir my senior year at Great Bend. I was always a pretty good singer and was selected to represent Great Bend in Wichita as a member of the Kansas (KMEA) State Choir. We spent a few days in Wichita and ended it with a concert which was recorded. I couldn't afford to buy a copy of the record and we didn't get them free, so I never had a chance to listen to it. But, the experience at the time was big stuff.

I was always a fish out of water in western Kansas even if I didn't fully understand it. I knew the day I left to go to college I would never be back to the sticks except to visit. I had nothing but scorn for those six years, but I also fully realized that it made me the person I had become – *extremely* individualistic – and one who really didn't need anyone else. Whether that's good or bad is a function of how you look at it.

And, looking at it from the perspective of committing suicide at age 60, my independent nature is probably why I found myself in this position in the first place. Perhaps if I had continued to be raised in a neighborhood with hundreds of other kids in Topeka, maybe my development would have been different. I don't blame my parents. I'm not sure I fit in all that well even when I was in Topeka. Presumably, it's all about genetic wiring. Barbie, and to a slightly lesser degree Mike, adapted much better than I did in western Kansas.

When I was a senior at Great Bend, I met with a math counselor who was visiting from Kansas State. He asked me specifically what I wanted to do. I told him I wanted to keep track of statistics – "You know, like football and basketball stats." He shook his head and said "If that's all you want to do, you might as well major in English!"

I never forgot that comment because I always considered *English and literature an absurd waste of time* – at least beyond high school. He tried to get me to consider advanced mathematics or physics or engineering. I told him I only wanted to do one thing. As it turns out, I took my share of math courses and quickly learned that computers were at least as interesting. Even so, no matter what else I learned about and liked, nothing ever compared to "keeping stats".

I spent most of my adult life in small business. However, every opportunity I had to employ statistical data, I did. Of course, back then it was before the kind of internet and computer tools we have nowadays. With the tools available by 2013, I was capable of spending 16 hours a day on statistical research, writing and analysis – and often did.

My Thoughts

We often find traumatic events in the childhoods and adolescence of those who die by suicide, but there is no severe trauma in Martin's early years. However, his family is not typical. His mother was an unplanned (accidental) baby, and his father was adopted. Both were only children. They had three children, but Martin does not describe a close family with love felt and shown between the family members. It sounds as if his family was an emotionally cold family, and it is interesting that none of the three children have had children themselves.

Martin was a middle child, the sibling position that is often the most neglected. The first-born is special, and often the first-born has the greatest need to achieve and does so. The last born is often spoilt. Even though Martin's parents were apparently cold individuals, these differences in the way children in different sibling positions are treated may have been present in a minimal way. The parents worked long hours (the mother at nights), so they were gone from the home much of the time.

Martin did have culture shock at the move to a rural town, and he adapted by becoming independent, *individualistic* in his words. He had few friends in middle or high school, although he did make one good friend with whom he remained friends for life. He became interested in sports and in statistics, hobbies which he eventually made use of in his career.

Martin's early years were, therefore, not overly traumatic, but his family is odd for want of a better word, One can see how those early years resulted in a Martin who, at the age of 60, lives alone, runs a sport website (an isolated job, sitting at a computer), and pondering when and how to die.

Chapter 14

OMG I Look 60

I not only *look* 60, I *think* 60. I *act* 60... I *am* 60!

I suspect most of us think we look younger than we really are. I know I did. I'm not exactly sure how I managed to avoid looking in the mirror the last 10-15 years. I *thought* I looked in the mirror, but either I didn't or else when I did, I saw only what I *wanted* to see. The sad reality is that my blindness must be related to vanity.

Now, that I can picture my head with a hole in it, I'm content to see myself at my *real* age. And, part of the reason is because I'll never have to see myself at 70 or 80 - and that's a good thing. And, every time I read that last sentence in the proofreading process, I get a smile on my face!

I thought I should find a place on this site to mention Fedoras. When I was about 54, I started wearing a Fedora all the time. Ok, I didn't wear one when I slept at night and I didn't wear one in church. Otherwise, 100% of the time - even when home alone. They just became part of who I was. There are plenty of people whom I've met over the past six years and have gotten to know that have never seen me without one.

At first, I just owned a couple of Fedoras, but then I bought a couple more. And, then I guess I got infected by the female shopping gene because, despite being extremely cheap, I got up to about a dozen hats. I finally stopped at 25 when I realized I wasn't going to be around in another 14 months (June 11, 2012). Besides, I had just about covered all the colors.

Don't think I paid a lot, though. I *did* buy a couple of them for about $20, but most were in the $10 range and a few were under $5 on close-out. I would guess my entire cost was $200 or so. But, I confess it was an indulgence of sorts, so I thought I would flash a picture of myself donning a Fedora for the site. And, while I'm at it, a pile of my collection - just before I donated them.

One thing is for sure, Fedoras may have caught my eye as a fashion statement, but shoes certainly never did. I bought a pair of hush puppy type shoes in 2001. They look like suede leather - gray. They were the most comfortable shoes I ever owned and although I only wore them once or twice a week for a few years, eventually, I wore them every day. I would estimate that I've worn those shoes at least 2,000 times. What kind of shoe could withstand 2,000 wearings? I can answer that... a $12 Earth Shoe from Wal-Mart!

But, shoes weren't the only thing I was cheap about. Take a look at my billfold. I had this puppy attached to my butt for the last 23 years of my life! I super-glued it back together on multiple occasions.

It became somewhat of a cold slap in the face when I realized that I had *become* my shoes... that I had *become* my billfold.

My Thoughts

All we learn from this brief entry is that Martin does not like getting old. (Who does?) And that he considers himself to be cheap.

Chapter 15

Mom and Dad

I discuss some issues related to my parents in the category "Growing Up" to the left side, but this will be more comprehensive and will include a few pictures. More pictures can be found under the category called... wait for it... "Pictures".

Francis Collins Manley (B: 11-23-23, D: 1-16-07, Age 83).

I take after my dad more than my mom. That's probably normal for a son, but you never know. My dad was never sick, my mom often was. I discussed in the category "Health" the fact that I barely know what being sick even means. I remember him having months of sick time built up that he never took. He worked for the Barton County Welfare Department in Great Bend, Kansas. When he left there, I believe he was paid for all those unused sick days.

He then went to work where my mom worked – Larned State Hospital. That was after the kids had all left home. My parents moved from about 15 miles from Larned into town.

My dad was also somewhat introspective. He read a lot. He told me once his IQ was 138. So, he was pretty smart. I suspect if computers had been around in his day, he would have gravitated to them just as I did.

The one major difference between us is that he loved to read. He read constantly and he could read *extremely* fast. He used to point out that he could read a major novel in a couple hours. It would take me a couple weeks if I did nothing else! That's why I never did it - duh! As a speed reader, he was constantly checking books out of the library and even worked at the Topeka Public Library before we moved to western Kansas. In his final years in Larned, Kansas, he actually taught a speed reading class at the Larned Public Library.

I'm not ashamed to admit that the only book I read through high school was Shag: The Last of the Plains Buffalo - a book for second graders. In fact, I was always kind of proud of it because I could say I bluffed my way through high school simply by reading the book jackets and asking my dad what it was about.

That subjective aspect of reading and, thus comprehending, is something that always turned me off. As a rule in life, the more subjective something was, the less I wanted to have anything to do with it. The more objective and verifiable, the more I was drawn to it.

Reading is such a bore unless it contains a lot of statistical data. I realize most people would say exactly the opposite, but I'm not most people, another duh. And, although I was a lot like my dad in many respects, I wasn't in the same hemisphere with respect to reading.

My dad was adopted and an only child. He had a birth certificate that he dug up somehow that showed his birth name to be Dallas Herman Ludwig and that his mother was a teacher. He was born in Kansas City. I searched for a long time hoping to uncover his birth family, but to no avail. Apparently, he had a German mother or father or both.

He grew up in Burlington, Kansas. He was dirt poor and had no prospects for employment when he graduated from high school. So, he went into the service. But, considering he graduated in 1941 – the same year Japan bombed Pearl Harbor, it was inevitable that he would be in the service one way or the other. He never advanced beyond Private First Class, but he fought for our country through World War II – spending his entire time in the Pacific theater. And, for that, he deserves respect.

He was in the Army, so although he traveled via ship from place to place, most of his time was on the ground – much of it in battle. He really didn't like to go into detail, but I remember him telling me about his best friend getting shot in the head – a fellow named "Lance". I also remember seeing (although I don't know whatever happened to it) a Japanese flag with a hole in each corner and blood stains around each hole. He told me it was folded into fourths and that he shot the guy. I guess it was common to take things off the dead Japanese soldiers and he had this flag under his shirt. It was a reminder of just how real is war.

After WWII, my dad used the GI Bill to go to college. He eventually graduated from Washburn University in Topeka with a degree in history - something he was incredibly proud of.

Unlike me, my dad didn't have a lot of idiosyncrasies – or if he did, he wasn't as obvious about them. My mom and dad didn't have a lot of other friends. My dad was perfectly content to come home from work to his house out in the middle of nowhere and sit in his easy chair and read, read, read.

Bertha Marie Hartzell (B: 8-28-26, D: 6-20-02, Age 77)

My mom was 15 years younger than the next youngest child in her family. Consequently, she grew up as an only child much like my dad. Her two brothers and two sisters were more like aunts and uncles to her and their kids (her nieces and nephews) were more like her cousins. As a result, we didn't know the rest of her family all that well even though we grew up in Topeka where her family was. But, when we moved to western Kansas (I was 11 going on 12), most of the contact with her family dried up - especially considering her parents had died either before I was born or very shortly thereafter.

My mom actually worked multiple jobs most of the time, which included a full-time job at Larned State Hospital as some kind of an aide. For many years she also sold Avon products. In fact, I remember her winning awards for most sales in some geographical area. She was relatively outgoing, but other than whoever she knew at LSH or via Avon or church, I'm not sure I remember her (or my dad) having friends – at least not the way I think of friends. I can't remember ever having another couple or another family over to our house.

Part of the reason might be that she was either working or sleeping and so there wasn't a lot of time to keep the house up or to entertain. My mom worked nights at LSH while my dad worked days either at Barton County Welfare or LSH. They didn't see each other much and we didn't see both of them together much. It was a very dysfunctional family for those days. Nowadays, big deal. What family isn't dysfunctional in some way?

My mom had stomach problems most of her adult life. It seemed like she was sick relatively often. I don't remember much of those days, so I can't put it in context except that compared to my dad who was never sick, it seemed like she was sick a fair amount. Even so, it didn't keep her from working all the time. And when she slept, it probably wasn't more than 4-6 hours.

She was also a huge country music fan. I don't know what caused that. Maybe she had a head injury as a child. Maybe she just liked the shape of a banjo. Who knows? Either way, she was so obsessive about it that we would work any kind of trip we were taking as a family around some concert somewhere. I remember Shreveport, Louisiana, for some inexplicable reason. I hated country music so bad that I refused to go into the concert. By this time I was probably 15 years old. So, I stayed in the car the entire time.

My mom became aware of my dad while he was in the war. I'm not sure how. She began writing to him and when he was discharged, they quickly met, dated and eventually got married on June 3, 1946. We celebrated their 50th anniversary in Larned in 1996.

The one thing I remember about my parents' later life was a love affair with girls' high school basketball in Larned... which was kind of strange. Here is this couple that didn't raise kids in Larned, didn't raise kids to play basketball and now were huge supporters of girls' basketball. Why not boys? Why not football?

My mom and dad were so passionate that they would actually travel to see the girls play. When your average opponent is 50 miles away and the sport is played during the winter, that's a *big* deal for an elderly couple. Their commitment to the program did not go unnoticed. On Friday, January 8th, 1999 they were honored during a home high school basketball game for their loyalty.

In the following Wednesday Larned *Tiller and Toiler* newspaper, there was a large picture of them receiving the plaque along with a very nice write-up.

There are sports fans, and then there are Mr. and Mrs. Francis Manley. Mr. and Mrs. Manley, no matter what the weather, have been loyal and faithful Larned High School sports boosters. Because of their loyal following, they were recipients of a special award during halftime of the Larned-Hoisington boy's basketball game Friday evening at the middle school gymnasium. "The Kansas State High School Activities Association made available an award to present to people in a community that exhibit loyal fan support and good sportsmanship," explained Larned High School Student Council Advisor Janet Fleske. The Larned High School Student Body, on behalf of the entire Larned High student body, then presented the Manley's with a beautiful plaque. "This evening the student body is proud to honor Mr. and Mrs. Francis Manley for their faithful support of school activities," said Larned High Student Council President Stacy Zook. "It doesn't matter what the weather is outside or how far it is to travel, we can always count on them to be at all of our games." "So, it is a great honor now for me to be able to present you with this plaque which reads: 'In Appreciation for your loyal dedication to Larned High School Athletics.' Thank you again for all of the support that you have shown us all of these years."

The *Tiller and Toiler* is the local newspaper and I used to call it the *Tillet and Toilet*, so when they were pictured in the paper, I just couldn't resist telling them that they finally got their mugs in the toilet. Bada Boom! I'll be here all week.

My mom has been deceased for over 11 years, my dad for over six. No parent should ever see a child die!!! It's just wrong on every level. If my parents were still alive – irrespective of how close we were as a family, I would never consider suicide. But, they won't know the difference.

We had each of them cremated. When my dad died, we were able to bury the ashes of both my mom and dad at the Leavenworth National Cemetery along with military honors. I kept a small amount of ashes from each and put them in heart-shaped jars. I filled them with blue stones for my dad and pink stones for my mom. I thought that was probably unique - and in some ways it certainly was. But, when I was pre-paying for my own cremation, I saw some very small urns on a shelf and asked the person what they were for. He said sometimes people save a small amount of the ashes and keep them in small urns. I felt a lot better about doing it myself after that.

My Thoughts

Martin calls his family dysfunctional, but I don't think it is. There was no abuse and no neglect. His mother worked long hours and was sick a lot, and his father read a lot. It is noteworthy that his father and mother had few friends. *I can't remember ever having another couple or another family over to our house.* Martin also does not remember his parents together much, except they did go to country music concerts and, in old age, to the high school girl's basketball games. So his father and mother were not alienated from each other.

The most noteworthy item is that, if his parents were alive, Martin would not have chosen suicide. His suicide would have caused his parents grief, and he would not want that. That is one of Marsha Linehan's reasons for living – responsibilities to family. – and it hints of some affection for his parents. Martin may feel distant from his family, but he has no anger and holds no grudges against them – and maybe he has some affection. He even kept some of their ashes in blue and pink jars!

Chapter 16

The Heavens

In 1965, our family moved from Topeka, Kansas to western Kansas, and even then, we were isolated far out in the countryside (coordinates = 38.377324, -99.01399). The one thing you could count on for at least a minimal amount of entertainment was... the sky. I can remember times when it was pitch black – no moon. You couldn't see your hand in front of your face, but you could see the stars! Boy, could you see the stars.

One other thing you could see was *shooting* stars. I don't recall whether that was a nightly occurrence, but I think it was. Obviously, some nights were more active than others. Of course, in the 1960's, I'm not sure they (astronomers) could tell you ahead of time when there would be shooting star shows. Nowadays, they know ahead of time for every location on the planet. For me at least, it was just guesswork and random luck.

For six years, that was a nightly form of entertainment in a place where there wasn't anything else. We had a 12" black and white TV and could only get two stations – two of the three major networks at the time. I believe one was in Hays, Kansas and one in Hutchinson, Kansas. We were pretty much in the middle between the two and the reception stunk. Simply put, we were isolated in the middle of nowhere – seemingly just a few miles from being off the edge of the world.

The house we lived in was actually a parsonage for a country church which was no longer being used as a church. It was locked and empty. Once I recall a wedding being held there, but otherwise it was vacant. A few years after we moved into the parsonage, some people came and picked up the entire church and moved it to Great Bend – about 13 miles away. They then filled in the basement with dirt and my dad used it as a garden for years.

The church – which was Lutheran – can now be seen on the south side of Great Bend, Kansas. It's part of an historical site and museum. The coordinates for it are 38.349633, -98.765523. You can view it via Google maps.

Before they moved it, my brother and sister and I used to lay out on the front porch of the church and look at the stars. It was sort of the ideal place because it was elevated concrete and it enabled us to avoid bugs. I remember once believing that I watched a star moving along the sky (which I suppose could have been an airplane), but then it stopped. I have very high spatial orientation abilities, so I noted where the "star" stopped relative to other stars. I remember watching for a long time and it never moved again. I remember looking up hundreds of times over my life and seeing the same star in the same location (duh). Obviously, I didn't see what I thought I saw, but it's something that always stuck with me.

So, the sky was our canvas and imagination our brush. Such is the life of city kids suddenly transplanted into the middle of the sticks.

I took astronomy in college and was surprised how much math was involved – and even though I'm very good at math, how difficult the course was. Nevertheless, I learned a lot and it made me all the more interested in the stars.

Considering how often you hear it now, it's hard to imagine anyone would not know how many stars are in the sky. There are roughly 200-400 billion (with a "B") stars in our galaxy – The Milky Way. But, the more amazing stat is that there are 100-200 billion *galaxies* in the *universe*. That makes the number of stars almost beyond comprehension.

One way to think of it would be to consider each person on earth to be a star. If so, there are about 6,400 billion times that many stars in the universe. So, for every single human, there are over six trillion solar systems out there – each with its own planets.

And, that's just what we know of. Our ability to see to the edges of the universe is limited. Of course, we dare not ask how many *universes* there are.

The magnitude of this expanse is one of the reasons why I was always fascinated with Sci-Fi movies (Star Trek and Star Wars series) and why I was a big fan of the TV series Star Trek: The Next Generation and Star Trek: Voyager. Just as when I was lying on my back in the middle of nowhere staring at the sky, it was a form of escapism.

One day when shopping with my family in 2001, I was in a store that had a lot of odd gadgets. One of them was a piece of electronics called "Night Navigator". It was later given to me by my second wife (Teri) as a present. This was a device that would mimic *your* sky at any given time.

You would set your latitude and longitude as well as the time and date. Then, by aiming it north and holding it in a fixed location, you could see your sky at that very moment by looking at the Night Navigator. Of course, seeing the sky was free, but the Night Navigator was a couple hundred bucks as I recall. What *it* offered that the *sky* did not was outlines of constellations along with the names. And, of course, the names of the planets and stars were also included. You could simply hold the Navigator up and then move your eyes to the sky to see what you otherwise would think was nothing more than a bunch of stars.

It was a great learning device and still would be if not for the fact that nowadays, there are free computer sites that do the same thing. You can take your tablet outside and accomplish exactly the same experience as the Navigator without it costing a cent. Here is one example.

Oddly enough, I think my fascination with the sky has always made me *more* confident of my religious beliefs though I also know that a relatively *small* number of astronomers and cosmologists believe in God (reportedly 7.5%) – at least the Judeo Christian God. For most of them, I suspect finding a relationship between trillions of stars and a book on earth (Bible) that claims to explain the creation of the universe is preposterous. They feel that if God *does* exist, he couldn't possibly care about us while he is governing this whole huge universe. I can understand that logic if an astronomer has no faith. However, for me, it's more evidence – if not *proof* – that God *must* exist. How else can it be explained? In view of the fact that I have only one "God option", I choose to believe that option. And, that seems pretty logical and scientific to me.

My Thoughts

Martin believes in God! How will he justify his choice of suicide given this?

Chapter 17

My Religion

Even though there are many reasons why I might not have committed suicide, the reasons to do it were superior. Having said that, the single biggest reason (by a mile) not to do it is because suicide is considered a mortal sin by many religions and I can't fault the logic.

Christianity is predicated upon the idea that anyone – no matter who they are and what they have done – can be reborn. And, that can happen at any time in their life – even minutes before death. It's also true that faith in God and trusting that he will guide your life is the fundamental guiding principle behind Christianity. Therefore, if the last thing you do before death is to *not* trust God, I can see where the ramifications might be just as *dire* as they would be *wonderful* when accepting Christ on one's deathbed.

So, how can I justify committing suicide. Here's a hint… I can't.

I'm a sinner. I will have sinned to the day I died. I've tried hard to be a better person the closer I got to the end, but I never wavered for a single second on my decision to take my own life – a decision I made on June 11, 2012. I took communion just before I died, taped this cross in my left hand and I asked God to forgive me. That's all I could do.

But, whether I could have done something more or something different, who knows? I did what I did. I decided that there simply was no way on this planet that I was going to be vulnerable in my old age! I wasn't going to *hope* someone would relieve my pain or come to see me when I was alone. I wasn't going to take a chance of ever running out of money or living in stress. I wasn't going to be exposed to people laughing at me or taking advantage of me. I did what I did because I was still on top at age 60, but lacked any confidence that I would be for much longer.

Whether or not it was God's will for me to do this is impossible for me to know. I would say it is impossible for *you* to know as well, but one thing about religion, people seem to *know* what seems impossible to know. Thus, the only thing I can say is that I appreciate your prayers despite your conviction and even though I have passed on.

It's also my hope that this web-site will be more than just a memorial to my life and those around me. That somehow, someway, it will be an inspiration – not to leave life prematurely, but to have a more *fulfilling* life and one that centers more around others than oneself. If I could bottle the last 14 months and apply it to a much earlier age, I would have been a far superior contributor to society!

I can say without fear of contradiction that since June 11, 2012, I have been much more focused on others than myself. I've done many things that I otherwise would not have done solely based upon the fact that I was not going to be around much longer and wouldn't have many more opportunities. Knowing it was coming to an end helped me focus on what was most important.

Consequently, my reasons for committing suicide include being able to help others financially. Whether that's a justifiable reason in your eyes, what can I say? Additionally, I became a better person. I looked for opportunities to have a positive influence on others – something I didn't do nearly enough before the last 14 months.

To the left side of this page, you will see categories for *Living Donor* and *Victory O Lord*. I decided late in 2012 that I wanted to donate a kidney before my death and I produced and distributed a number of pictures of Moses (Victory O Lord) to various churches and organizations. I hope you will read both of those stories. I also grew my hair out until it was long enough to donate to cancer patients. Trust me, I hated having long hair, but it was something I could do that was positive and so I did. I also gave away a lot of personal possessions to a Catholic charity.

Knowing when is your last day on Earth is *amazingly* liberating. It places a sense of urgency upon all that you do. It removes the fog of a complicated life and worries about the future. It makes you prioritize as you probably should have all along. Consequently, it provides more satisfaction than one might otherwise have. Although, it simply would not have been possible to do all the things I've done in the last 14 months for all the months of my life before that, I realize how much more I *could* have done! *Believing* I should is one thing, but *doing* what I should do is another.

As James says… "What does it profit, my brethren, if a man says he has faith, but has not works? Can his faith save him? If a brother or sister is ill-clad and in lack of daily food, and one of you says to them, 'Go in peace, be warmed and filled,' without giving them the things needed for the body, what does it profit? So faith by itself, if it has no works, is dead." (James 2:14-17) His point continues on through the 26th verse.

I was born in a Christian home and raised in a Christian church. As I mentioned in other places on this site, I got away from organized religion around the age of 30 and didn't reenter it until the age of 45. Whether in or out, I've been a sinner and I'm ashamed of my actions. However, as a Christian, I know that I have been granted grace by the sacrifice of Christ. That's the premise we live by. Intellectual assent, however, is not enough. As James goes on to say… "Even the demons believe – and shudder."

Not many people know this about me, but when I was 22 years old, I began memorizing the Bible. The way I did it was that I began with the book of James and the first verse. I repeated it all day long until I had said it to myself 100 times or more. The next day, I learned the second verse. I repeated both verses together a 100 times. The third day, I did the same thing and on and on and on. For a year and a half, I memorized a new verse each day. At least once every day, I repeated the entirety of what I had memorized. Of course, I had a young brain back then. I could barely do three verses in a month today!

Still, it was an impressive endeavor. I memorized the book of James, then Colossians, then 1st Peter, then the first five chapters of Matthew and the first three chapters of 1st Timothy. At that point, I was nearing 500 versus. It wasn't a problem to add a verse each day and it wasn't like I could forget all the verses I'd learned. After all, I had repeated them every single day. However, the problem was that I was running out of time – meaning it was harder and harder to recite the entirety of what I had memorized each day because it took so long. I realized I couldn't do that indefinitely and as obsessive as I was about the process, it scared me into believing that someday I simply would no longer be able to remember every verse I had learned because I wouldn't have time to repeat the entirety every day. I'm such an all-or-nothing type person that it caused me to just stop cold. I got through the third chapter of 1st Timothy and the final verse which reads...

> "Great indeed, we confess, is the mystery of our religion: He was manifested in the flesh, vindicated in the Spirit, seen by angels, preached among the nations, believed on in the world, taken up in glory." (1st Timothy 3:16)

Not a bad verse to end with! Even though the experience ended at 497 versus and 497 days, it was rewarding and it has always meant that the book of James had a special place in my heart because that's the one I began with and the one I repeated over and over every day along the way.

Thus, it always gnawed at me that James makes a major issue out of the distinction between intellectual assent and practicing faith. I've just never led my life as one should who is truly faithful. That is, as I said at the top of this section, the real issue when it comes to ending one's life – a lack of (enough) faith.

So, I hope nobody will read this site and be motivated into committing suicide. This site is not here to justify it and it's not here for that reason. Besides, how many people are like me in this world? Maybe two if I'm looking in a mirror.

Instead, my hope is that anyone reading this will recognize that I have mixed emotions and mixed logic with respect to how I reconcile my Christianity with suicide. But, I've really never strayed from the fact that I believe in Christ and I believe the story of the Bible.

How do I know God exists? I know because I know. That's about the most concrete answer any Christian can give. I realize it doesn't make for good debate, but then most matters of the heart and mind are *subjective* to one person, but *objective* to another.

I do not believe the Earth is 6,000 years old. That's pure nonsense in my opinion. There was a time when I was very young that I *did* believe it. I started with Genesis and tracked the lineage of each person. The one thing I discovered - and at the time it meant a great deal to me - was that the last living recorded person in the Bible at the time of the flood - except Noah and his family - was Methuselah. He was the oldest person to live according to the Bible at 969 years of age. But... it just so happens that he died the year of the flood.

Methuselah was 187 years older than Lamech. Lamech was 182 years older than Noah. Therefore, Methuselah was 369 years older than Noah. So, when Noah was 600 (the year of the flood), Methuselah was 969 (his age at death) and Lamech died five years earlier. It would have been contradictory had anyone still been living based upon their age *after* the flood since everyone died (we are told) except Noah and his family.

Nevertheless, it didn't take much exposure to science to realize the Earth wasn't 6,000 years old. It's millions and hundreds of millions – even billions of years old. Evolution is something that no intelligent person can deny. How it plays exactly into the Bible story and Christianity is something I cannot answer. Nevertheless, just as God allows humans to evolve from babies to adults, I see no problem with assuming that he would allow humankind the ability to evolve as well.

We, as intelligent human beings, know that the Sun is one of 300 billion stars just in our galaxy. Our galaxy is one of 170 billion galaxies in the known Universe. It's complete insanity to believe we are the only living creatures in the Universe. There is a better chance in my opinion that you could travel to anywhere in Florida at random, go to any shoreline you wanted, pick up any grain of sand you choose and that I would be able to guess which grain of sand it was. By all scientific accounts, the development of life on Earth is incredibly unique and unbelievably unlikely. The number of things that had to happen in order for life to develop is so remote, it might as well be a miracle. Therefore, I don't see it as a stretch at all that God created the miracle we call Earth. And, if so, I don't see it as odd that he would want to populate it with living creatures and that there would be a logical hierarchy and that he would want some kind of interaction with the top of the order. But, God is God and who am I? Even so, as a human being, it seems reasonable. How humans became humans is probably less about Adam and more about evolution. But, that still doesn't mean God didn't make it happen. Even though there are almost certainly billions of other planets in the Universe that have life and almost certainly millions of them that have life which is vastly more advanced than our own, that doesn't mean God didn't create the Universe and the Earth... and you.

There was a time when mankind thought the Sun revolved around the Earth. The presumption was that humans were the center of the Universe. Today, we know we are not. Thus, why should Earth be unique among the heavens? If there is an entity that created the Universe – and I can't see any argument against it – then it stands to reason God could have made the Earth and millions of other inhabitable planets in the Universe – all of which may have had a unique experience with God – maybe the same God, maybe not. After all, if one believes in God and believes God made Earth for his pleasure for His interaction, then it defies common sense that He would have stopped with just one planet in this massive incomprehensible universe.

The way I look at it is that any God big enough to create the Earth and the life therein is a big enough God for me to be satisfied there need be no others - so it really doesn't matter if there are a million or a billion or a trillion inhabitable planets out there. It will be forever before we can travel to our closest star. I'm not a believer in bending space and negating the limitations of the speed of light. So, from my perspective, our "universe" is our *solar system* and always will be. I don't need to be concerned about what God has done outside of it. Nevertheless, the evidence is overwhelming that whatever force created our solar system has created trillions of other solar systems. And, as unlikely the probabilities of life on Earth, it's still all but a mathematical certainty that life exists on millions of other planets.

It's ironic, I suppose, that the Christian basis for believing in God is faith and faith is hard to prove. However, the evidence for believing that there must be a God is *scientifically* proven IMO because nothing but God could have created the Universe.

I pray that God will forgive me and through his grace via the sacrifice of his Son, I will be saved.

My Thoughts

Many people change their religious views when they choose suicide. They convince themselves that God will understand their choice. In case God does not, they ask others to pray for them, hoping that those prayers will have an impact. Some turn away from religion. But not Martin. He believes, and he knows that suicide is considered to be a sin in his religion. He prays himself to God for forgiveness. He took communion on the day before he died and taped a cross to his left hand. Many religious people focus on reunion with deceased parents and other significant others after they die by suicide, but Martin does not have appear to have any reunion fantasies.

He again talks of the fear of old age, especially declining and dying *alone*. Living alone was tolerable for Martin, but declining and slowly dying alone is not tolerable. His turning outward, his altruism, is a new theme. His life was not fulfilling, he believes, because he was too self-centered. He should have concerned himself more with others. He has tried to make up for this a little in his last months by being altruistic –helping others financially (as will his death with his life insurance and any money he leaves in his will), donating his organs, giving away his possessions to a Catholic charity, and donating his long hair.

His fear of dementia and death, however, outweighs what he could do for others and his belief in God.

Chapter 18

Chancel Choir

As I've mentioned elsewhere on this blog, I've been a singer all my life. But my only real experience in recording anything was when I was a senior in high school in 1971 and I was selected to the KMEA State Choir in Wichita. We made a record, but I wasn't able to get a copy because it cost $5 or whatever it was at the time – and we were poor.

Though I'm pretty sure my best days as a singer were before I was 47 years old, that's when I joined the Chancel Choir at Advent Lutheran Church in Olathe, Kansas. The year was 2000 and it coincided with the opening of our new sanctuary.

Tom Williams is one of my heroes in life and he works tirelessly to run the music program for the church. He's also the choir director. The choir has around 35 members on average from year to year. The average age is probably 50 and we may average 25-27 singers for any given Sunday performance – factoring in the many other responsibilities people have.

I've always thought our choir was exceptionally good. I'm 100% positive I'm biased, but there are other pieces of evidence – which include the praises of non-members. It's been a joy to be part of it all these years. We also produced three CDs (see below). I doubt if anyone will read this and order copies, but I think they can still be had. Just go to *Advent's* website and pick up the phone or send an email.

I sang in choir in high school and I sang bass. I was recruited to sing in Advent's Chancel Choir by a tenor (Lloyd) and so I sang tenor for around nine years. I never really liked the tenor part, although the range wasn't a problem. It was just not as easy for me to find the notes as it was the bass part. Plus, the other problem was that during all those years – or at least most of them - the tenors weren't really in one spot. We had a couple on the front row, a couple on the second row and several in the third row. I sat in the front row and most of the tenors around me were weak singers - *good* singers, but they didn't have strong voices. The other parts around me were more dominant and I had to overcome them to learn my part. I have a pretty strong voice, but I really didn't feel like I could sing tenor with much confidence compared to how I later felt singing bass.

About four years ago, I switched to bass and loved it. It's really where I wish I had been all those years. The other advantage is that the basses are on the end and I was on the end of the basses – meaning about all I could hear were other basses and almost all of them have strong voices. I was in a far better place to simply sing my part. Besides, although the range of a tenor was doable, the older I got the more I didn't enjoy straining my voice for long periods of time singing higher notes. Thus, the move to bass enabled me to really enjoy my final years in the choir.

I never liked using anymore brain cells than absolutely necessary and so I was always disappointed when we *had* to learn new music. Of course, once we learned it and added yet another song to our repertoire, I was glad we did it. So, it was kind of a catch-22.

Every so often Tom would introduce a new piece and we would collectively dislike it enough that we would find a way to get him to forget about it. On several occasions, someone would yell out something to the effect of "I've got $20 to ban this piece of music." Someone else would yell out "I've got $20.", and so forth. Ok, maybe the "someone" was most often me. I can remember Tom collecting a couple hundred bucks for the choir fund just to avoid having to learn a particular song. He missed the boat, however. He should have intentionally tried to make us learn some really bad songs just to raise money.

Ultimately, over my 13 years in the choir, we learned and sang at least 100 songs and possibly as many as 150. In the last couple years, we have gravitated toward re-singing many of those we already know - or at least *knew*. I always felt that unless it was a song we sang all the time - and there were only a handful of those - that the congregation wouldn't mind us singing songs we had sung in the past for the simple reason that 1) they may not have worshipped at Advent when we last sang it, 2) they may not have been at that service and 3) who can remember one song years before? Thus, the last couple years were the best years of all for me and my tiring brain.

A reasonably big part of why I opted for suicide was in watching a member of our choir (who was about my age) deteriorate before our eyes. Frank was/is a good guy, but over a period of half dozen years, his brain abandoned him and he couldn't function on his own. It was pathetic. Eventually, he ended up in a nursing home when he was younger than me. I knew as I watched Frank that I would be him someday and I also knew that I would never let that happen in a million years! As I got closer and closer to becoming Frankish, I realized my day was near. So, although there were many reasons that led me to this decision, none individually was bigger than seeing what happened to Frank. Poor guy!

Over the years we took a number of trips to churches in the Kansas City area and even a few several hours away in Kansas. It was always a joy to be able to share the gift of song with other congregations even if it was time-consuming.

Tom developed a new liturgy for our church. It's called Service of Joy and has a much more modern feel. I never belonged to, or even attended, a Lutheran church before 1998 when I moved to Overland Park, Kansas. I went because my wife-to-be (Teri) had been raised Lutheran and she attended the church. I never felt all that super comfortable with the Lutheran liturgy. I think that's something you are either raised with or it takes some getting used to. Certainly by 2013, I was comfortable, but most of the reason was the Service of Joy.

Tom introduced SOJ to the congregation around 2003. It seems much more applicable to this day and age than the old liturgies. Though it is more modern, SOJ doesn't in any way, omit the critical aspects of the Lutheran liturgy. It's just more melodic – a big *big* plus in my opinion. I can't imagine for the life of me why other churches would not adopt it for their worship services. But, it's pretty much a fact nowadays that all churches are different.

I lived in Florida for two months in the summer of 2004. When I was there, I went to a different Lutheran church every Sunday. What amazed me was how diverse they were. They had similarities to be sure, but that's like saying a brother and sister have similarities. They also have major differences. So, although SOJ has great potential, who can say what will happen with it outside of Advent?

More than simply singing in the choir, was the fact that being involved brought me back to my Christian roots. I was born and raised in a Christian household and I was part of a number of different religious groups until around the age of 30. Then, for about 15 years, I wasn't involved in any organized religion. When I moved to Overland Park, Kansas at the age of 45, I started going to Advent and never regretted the decision.

The value of a church depends upon how comfortable it makes a person feel. There are so many options today, it's difficult to know what people want and what they don't. About all any church can do is try to stay true to itself and hope that it has a formula that works for others. I always felt that our choir was a big part of what people in the congregation appreciated about Advent. I'm sorry I won't be part of it in the future, but it will continue on as strong as ever, at least until everyone else starts getting old – and that's not that far away for a lot of them.

Advent is buried deep in the suburbs of Johnson County, Kansas. *JOCO* is part of the metropolitan area for Kansas City. When the church began 30+ years ago, it was young and in a rapidly growing area. The population around Advent has become much more stabilized by now and Advent, as well as the choir, will need to be as current and relevant as it can be to attract new members. Personally, I think SOJ, as well as the kind of music the choir sings, are both strong reasons for others to worship there – and if they sing, participate in the choir.

Our choir took great pleasure in focusing on two primary composers. Naturally, we sang songs from dozens of composers over the years, but there were two that we felt exceptionally strong about – *Joe Martin* and *Pepper Choplin*.

I would classify both of them as musical geniuses. They have each visited our church on more than one occasion and we became as close to them as one can be for a composer halfway across the country. Neither are Lutheran, but so what? Their music is generic and applicable for any Christian service. There are a number of songs by each on our three CDs (see below).

There isn't a great deal more to say about my experiences in the choir. I love Tom and Janelle (our pianist) and the people that make up the choir. I'm proud to be able to say I was part of such a wonderful group for 13 years.

My Thoughts

Martin is writing this in the months before his death. Does he sound as if he has dementia? Not a bit! But the fear is there, especially when he sees colleagues (in the choir) succumb to senility. And we learn that he belonged to this group. He hasn't become a hermit. There are people in the choir whom he will miss.

Chapter 19

Victory O Lord

Back when I was 23 years old, I was in Manhattan, Kansas, at the public library and I saw a book of paintings. As I was flipping through the pages, I immediately focused in on a painting of Moses with his arms being held up by two men. I can't recall if I knew (or remembered) the biblical story at that moment, but if not, I soon learned of the story in Exodus 17:8-13.

I thought the picture was *amazing* – powerful and colorful, impressive in every way, though the image above just doesn't reflect that as well as it does if it is in front of you. Anyway, that was in 1976. Although I never forgot the picture, I also was no longer in Manhattan and unable to figure out what the picture was. It just remained a memory for over two decades. In those days (pre internet) it was like trying to find a needle in a haystack, had I even tried. If the internet was invented for only one reason, it was so that I could find this picture. Eventually, I did.

I discovered the picture was in a museum in Manchester, England. I contacted them and they sent me an 8x10 black and white. For several years, I had it in a frame, but I was never satisfied. I remembered the colors being striking and B&W just didn't cut it. Eventually, in 2005, I contacted the museum and ordered a 12x16 color print. When I got it, I found a great frame and took them both to a frame shop to have the mat produced and to have the whole thing put together for a final 16x20 picture. I hung it in my study for two years before I decided it needed to be seen by more than just me.

In 2007, I took it to the pastor of my church (Roger, Advent Lutheran, Olathe, Kansas) and offered to donate it. He appreciated the picture and since then, it has hung in the library at the church where it is to this day.

Once I realized I didn't have long to live, I decided that I wanted to give away more of these pictures. I ordered five more copies of Victory O Lord and had plaques made. I bought five more frames and took them all to the same frame shop. They put them together and I had what I considered to be five masterpieces.

Obviously, beauty is in the eye of the beholder and I can't expect anyone else to feel the exact same way about a picture. But, for me, it is the best religious painting ever created. To see it close up with the blazing colors is *really* special.

So, I sent out a few emails to various local churches – Catholic and Lutheran. I received back requests for the picture from one Lutheran church and two Catholic churches. I donated the pictures to those three churches along with my own. That left me with two pictures.

I decided I would like to have as much visibility as possible, so I contacted Rockhurst University in Kansas City and they were excited to get a copy. I then contacted the Jewish Community Center in Overland Park, Kansas. They were also very excited about it.

The plaque on the front at the bottom reads: "As long as Moses held up his hands the army of the Israelites prevailed; when he lowered them the enemy prevailed. As the battle raged on and Moses' hands grew weary, Aaron and Hur stood beside him and held up his hands so the army of Israel was victorious. (Exodus 17)

There is another plaque on the back that reads: Victory O Lord, John Everett Millais, 1871, Manchester Art Gallery, England, Donated by Martin Manley 2013. Of course, the plaque at my own church reads… Donated by Martin Manley 2007.

I'm not sure what value there is of this picture in a church school or library. I can only say that if anyone develops an appreciation for it and if it in any way deepens their faith, then it was worth the time, effort and money. I've never seen this picture anywhere else or even referred to by anyone, so I feel it remains mostly unknown. I have no idea why that would be the case except that it is from the Old Testament – and a good deal of modern-day Christianity barely acknowledges the OT except for Genesis and Psalms.

If you Google Victory O Lord, you will see numerous references to it, but they are all in context of who painted it and when. There just is no reference to who it inspired. At least now, there is one place on the web of someone who found it to be magnificent!

My Thoughts

This essay attests to Martin's religious beliefs and his generosity and altruism in his final months.

Chapter 20

The Proposal

There were times when I was actually a romantic – although even being romantic was tempered by my analytical way of thinking. But, in this particular case, that made what I did in my proposal to my second wife (Teri) special – at least in my opinion.

I knew I wanted to propose to her in May, 1999, but I got a great idea. I decided to do it via a crossword puzzle. She loved to work CW puzzles and I thought it would be cool.

Years later in 2011, I heard of a person who got a professional CW writer to create a puzzle specifically for him and they worked it into the paper. The three answers in the puzzle were marlowe epstein willyoumarryme. I'm not sure what the clue was for "marlowe" or "espstein", but it worked.

Mine was cooler in my opinion. We were taking a trip from May 28th to June 1st to the Ozarks in southern Missouri. I decided I wanted to propose on June 1st – the traditional first day of summer. June is also the month in which most weddings occur. May 28th was on a Friday and June 1st was on a Tuesday – which worked out perfectly.

Teri liked doing crossword puzzles because she was good at them. She was always smart – getting her degree and MBA while working full time – straight A's. She then got her CPA. She doesn't like me bragging on her and she will probably hate this category on this site, but what can she do about it now?

Anyway, I made up a crossword puzzle (see below) that I knew she would want to do. I made it the size of USA Today's paper and put it in as an insert on May 28th. We took off for the Ozarks on that Friday with me driving. At some point, I handed her the USA Today. She immediately discovered the insert and started working on it.

The theme of the crossword puzzle was "The Wedding Month" by Lyman Mintear (anagram for Martin Manley). It stated right on it that the answers would appear June 1, 1999.

I'm so obsessive about detail that I decided I had to make the crossword puzzle symmetrical, as all good CW puzzles are. Even cooler, the word "symmetry" is in the exact middle of the puzzle. Needless to say, that meant it took a lot of hours to create – especially when there was a theme and as many clues as possible had to relate in some way to love, romance, weddings, etc.

She completed the puzzle and then discarded it like she might with any other puzzle she worked on. Of course, when she got out of the car, I discretely saved it so that she would have it Tuesday to check the answers even if she didn't think of it herself.

When we got back to Overland Park, Kansas on June 1st and settled in, I bought a USA Today paper and put the new insert into it. The insert showed the puzzle filled in with the answers. The point was that she was supposed to fill in the answers to the clues above. When she did, they spelled out… T L W, W I L L Y O U M A R R Y M E? M A M. TLW were her initials and MAM were mine. Foolishly, she said "yes".

"My most brilliant achievement was my ability to be able to persuade my wife to marry me." -- Winston Churchill

Many of the answers to the puzzle were related to the theme - JUNEFIRST, SHE, ROMEOANDJULIET, SEX, LOVE, ENGAGEMENT, MARRY, LADY, HEART, BRIDEANDGROOM, SAYYES, WINEANDDINE, WOMEN, DESIANDLUCY, SUGARANDSPICE, RING, HERS, WED, IDO, AMORE, MOON, MAKEAWISH, BELLS and others.

My Thoughts

Martin married twice! This boy, who developed the habit of being a loner and spent his last few months writing two blogs (alone), married, twice in fact. Of course, he was also divorced twice. And he could be a romantic! Another surprise from what has gone before.

Chapter 21

Two Marriages

I have been married twice and there are various references to both wives and both marriages on this site apart from just this page. It's pretty hard to discuss one's life without discussing what it was like or what it meant to be married – especially when the total years of marriage were around 21 and half years.

I don't mean to imply 21.5 years of marriage is a great deal of time – especially since it's the sum of two marriages. By comparison, my parents were married 56 years when my mom passed away. Still, 20+ years in anyone's adult life is a long time and it covers a lot. First Chris and then Teri.

Chris: Married 3-28-81, Divorced 11-10-97

I first saw Chris in an evening Economics class at Washburn University in September, 1980. I had just gone back to school and I immediately zeroed in on her. Poor girl. Being relatively brave and having relatively little concern about what anyone else thinks, I followed her home one night after class. Once I knew where she lived, I think I waited a couple days and put a note on her windshield. Chris had a small house without a garage – just a carport.

I wrote my name and phone number on the note and told her that I had seen her in class and that for all I knew she had a boyfriend who would beat the hell of me. I asked only that if she was in a committed relationship (I didn't see a ring), that she just throw away the note. She could have saved herself by simply having a trash can nearby.

Instead she called me and we hit it off immediately. We were talking marriage within a few months. But, you have to recognize that I was 27 and she was 29 at the time. Both of us were to the point where we were ready to settle down. By early in 1981 we were setting the date at March 28th.

Our honeymoon was one for the ages and there is a separate category to the left specifically called "*Honeymoon...s*" under "Trips and Travel". Therefore, I won't go into that here.

When I met Chris, she had a dog named "Cleo" – an Old English Sheepdog. Cleo was a great pet – except that she ate a ton and was huge. But, I came to love her a lot and I spent a lot of time with her. Chris had a veterinarian already, of course, so when it came time to have her nails cut, we took her in to him. When she came back to us, her four paws were bandaged. Whoever cut the nails, cut them too short and they bled. Unfortunately, she would chew on her bandages, so we put one of those cone-shaped things around her neck to keep her from being able to put her mouth to her paws. Even so, within a matter of days, she was limping badly. Obviously, we didn't know what was wrong, so we took her back to the vet. He kept her a day or two and then called and told us that her bandages had been wrapped too tight and she had lost circulation in one of her paws and that the leg would have to be amputated! We were crushed, of course, but I gave him the go-ahead. The next day he called and said she died.

Apart from breaking up (or more aptly being broken up) with my first two girlfriends when I was in high school and college, that was the worst thing that had ever happened to me. If it were 10 years later and that happened, I would have made the vet's life a living hell, but at the time, I was still too young and not as ready to go after someone as I would have been later. If it happened today, of course, you could bury someone like that on the internet. But, it's just as well that it happened when it did. Revenge would have only been time-consuming.

Of course, we got over it as people always do. We got a small black dog named Samantha (Sammy) from the pound and went to a breeder and picked out another Old English Sheepdog puppy (Priscilla). Sammy was a great dog and we had her for a long time. Priscilla was problematic. Old English Sheepdogs are very active and hyper by nature. I, being the idiot I was, picked this dog from the litter because he was the one that wanted to chew on my shoe while the others seemed less interested. I should have chosen the one that was closest to being comatose, but I did just the opposite and we paid for it for years. I suggested getting rid of her many times, but Chris is a woman and... I think we all know what that means.

We had other cats and even another dog later on, but none of them could compare to Cleo, except Sammy.

We didn't take many vacations even though we had the money. I was just tight. I liked to put it in savings and invest. I was smart enough about numbers to recognize the *value* as well as the *curse* of compounded interest. I knew we could be millionaires and retire by the time we were 60 if we just were conservative about spending money. So, we were.

We bought a nice house in 1983 and I actually built two additions to it. But, that wasn't lost money. I got every cent out of it when I sold it in 1998. We didn't buy expensive cars although we bought a new car in 1985 and 1988. But, both were inexpensive small cars and we got lots of years out of them.

Overall, we were relatively conservative with money even though we both made a decent living. Consequently, we had a nice nest egg by the time we were ready to...~~retire~~...divorce.

Chris and I drifted apart. I take 100% of the blame. She was a very committed person and would do anything for me. It's not intended to be an excuse, but my mom and dad were essentially both an only child. They really didn't understand, nor were they able, to pass on the idea of "family". Both parents and my two siblings were all relatively individualistic people. We lived out in the sticks, many miles from the nearest town. You either learned how to entertain yourself or you would go crazy. I probably did a little of both as it turns out. But, one thing is for sure... I learned how to exist in my own world.

Unfortunately, that carried over to my marriage. Chris wanted children because 1) she's normal and 2) she came from a traditional family and extended family. I never did *not* want children, but I was never ready. I loved my friends' kids, but it was a totally different thing seeing them for an hour or two at a time versus being responsible for them 24/7/365 for life... and OMG... changing their diapers!

Careers just got in the way and so we would take different kids places – even on short trips over the weekend, but we never had kids of our own. I regret to this day that I took 16 years of Chris' life and she never had children. But, at the same time, I don't regret that *I* never had my own children. I would have loved them to death, but I'm not sure what the results of being a father would have been like.

As I stated, I wasn't raised in a "family" environment like most people. In one sense, the proof is that I was married twice and never had children. My brother has been married for over 20 years and never had children. My sister has been married over a long period of time and never had children. It's not rare for a couple to be childless, even if it's by their choice and not a health issue. But, it *is* rare for all three siblings to be childless by choice. I'm confident that it goes back to our situation where we basically fended for ourselves, especially in our teen years and we never really got the "family" thing.

> "I have learned that only two things are necessary to keep one's wife happy. First, let her think she's having her own way. And second, let her have it." -- Lyndon B. Johnson

Eventually, Chris and I led two completely different lives and it was only a matter of time before we got a divorce. I remained friends with Chris and have to this day. I tried to help her any way I could after our divorce.

Chris and I separated in May, 1997, but we didn't get a divorce until November. The divorce was amicable and we used the same attorney. I think she's forgiven me for whatever it was she needed to forgive me for.

COOL FACTOID: Both wives pursued their Bachelor's degrees and Master's degrees in business at Baker University.

Teri: Married 7-31-99, Divorced 6-3-04

After my divorce with Chris I wasn't interested in pursuing another relationship for a while, mostly because I had no way to meet anyone. I didn't go bar-hopping because I didn't drink. But, then I discovered Matchmaker on line. It didn't keep people from lying, but it was still a pretty good service.

I met a few women and had a few dates. But, then I made contact with Teri in early July, 1998. We began dating. She lived in south Johnson County, Kansas – which is the extreme southerly suburbs of Kansas City - about an hour from Topeka where I lived. I immediately fell in love with the area.

I had driven around in JOCO a few times before. It reminded me of Houston in 1973-75 when I lived there. Clean, new, modern, wealthy. I knew the schools were great and there was very little crime. I also knew that I wanted to live there someday.

I pretty much despised Topeka where I lived from ages 1-11 and 25-44. In 1960, Topeka had 120,000 people. Today, Topeka has about 127,000, although if you count the entire county, maybe 200,000. Nevertheless, there are good reasons it has barely grown. On the other hand, Overland Park, Kansas has grown from 21,000 in 1960 to 175,000 today! OP is the biggest city in JOCO, but the entire county is just one big suburb of 560,000. Anyway, that's where I wanted to be.

We were closing down the last company I had worked with in Topeka and I decided to sell my house and move. I sold the house on the first day it was on the market and before you could say "Goodbye Topeka", I had moved to Johnson County.

Teri and I dated through 1998 and 1999 and got married on July 31st, 1999.

The great thing about Teri was that she has two daughters – Jaime and Marissa who were eight and six at the time. They are both great kids. Jaime has since graduated Kansas State with a Masters in Accounting. She's taking her CPA this summer and already has a job beginning in the fall with a firm in KC. Marissa just completed her third year at K-State.

No matter how much I liked the idea of a second chance marriage – especially with kids, I was still largely a fish out of water. I tried to be moldable and God knows, Teri tried to mold me. But, at some point, I think I rebelled against it because I just felt I was losing my identity. In any event, we really weren't made for each other.

> "All marriages are happy. It's the living together afterward that causes all the trouble." -- Raymond Hull

That hasn't kept us from being friends – actually pretty good friends – in the nine years since we got divorced. We've done many dozens, if not hundreds, of things together and I've maintained as close a relationship as possible with the girls. I lived only about a mile away from Teri, so it was easy to be there for whatever she needed help with. The one thing I can feel okay about is that there is hardly an inch on that house that I didn't redo in the years during our marriage or after our divorce.

Teri isn't a spendaholic by any means, but nobody is cheap like me. At least, no woman. At least, no women in south Johnson County, Kansas! Consequently, that created some problems. I never wanted to go on vacations and spend the money – although we went a few places. But, mostly it was a clash of personalities and priorities. Once we were no longer required to *conform*, we were very content around each other.

I have no doubt whatsoever that both Teri and Chris are going to be shocked, if not devastated by what I've done. I'm sorry, but I did what I think is the best thing to do. Nobody can make that decision for me and I couldn't be concerned what anyone else's opinion might have been. *Nothing* was going to change my mind. I spent 14 months thinking about my suicide plan - probably 100 times a day - and I'm serious. I've thought it through like nobody has ever thought anything through. Will it break hearts? Of course, it will. But, you know what? It would have only been a matter of time before hearts were broken anyway. News flash... *Someday*, I was going to die!

I loved both Chris and Teri to the day of my death and I have great appreciation for the fact that there was a time when I was important enough to them to be a partner in life. It didn't work out and I take full responsibility in both cases. Nobody is to blame but me.

My Thoughts

Two marriages, and Martin takes the blame for their ending. In the first, their differences over having children drove a wedge between them. In the second, *we really weren't made for each other*. The divorces are unusual in that Martin remained good friends with both ex-wives. He has no anger toward either wife. He thinks that they will be shocked by the news of his suicide, but he is not close enough to either of them to discuss it with them. Both of them probably got e-mails that he says he sent prior to his suicide, but this may be the first time they knew of his suicidal intentions.

Chapter 22

First Two Loves

As I mentioned in *"Growing Up"* to the left, our family moved to western Kansas when I was 11 going on 12. We lived roughly nine miles north of a little town called Pawnee Rock which was about seven miles NE of Larned. My mom worked in Larned and eventually, so did my dad. As you can imagine, they had a few miles to drive every day.

My best friend was Charles and he lived near Larned and went to school there. We were friends because his dad and my dad worked together in Great Bend, but his dad was also the pastor of a small Christian Church that we went to in Pawnee Rock. Got all that?

From time to time as I got older, I would visit Charles and one late summer day while I was just about to enter my junior year at Pawnee Rock, Charles and I went to a church fellowship in Larned...

...My first love is named Lucinda Kay (Cindy).

Cindy was at this fellowship and it was the first time I had ever seen her. Both Charles and Cindy were a year older than I and in the same class at Larned - soon to be seniors. He decided he liked her. Near the end of evening, we gathered in a prayer circle. We were going to hold hands, so Charles quickly positioned himself next to Cindy. I was on his other side. The person running the meeting asked us to hold the hand of the person *two people* away from us! It meant I got hold Cindy's hand and, as irony would have it, we held hands right in front of Charles... SUCKER! One thing led to another and I got the guts to ask her out.

I can't begin to tell you how much I fell head over heels, but then that's common, I suppose, for a first love.

Even at that tender age, there was conflict between what a girlfriend might fear about how I was seen by others versus my not caring much - if at all. I can remember two examples. Once we were at a motel restaurant. I don't recall many people there. We were in a booth and we both had tea to drink. I opened about six packets of sugar and dumped them in the tea and began stirring it. She freaked out - and I'm confident it wasn't concern over my health. In retrospect, I can't even begin to imagine why someone would care (or be embarrassed) by how many packs of sugar another person put in their tea. Of course, I'm sure I've embarrassed dozens (if not *hundreds*) of people I was with at various times in my life. I was oblivious to most of it, but even if I knew I was an embarrassment... I wouldn't have cared. I'm sure I thought, or would have thought, that was *their* problem, not mine.

On another occasion, Cindy and I traveled to Manhattan (about three hours from the sticks) for some college preparation thing. By this time, my friend Charles had a girlfriend named Beth. I met some friends I knew from summer camps in Manhattan and on two separate occasions that day for some inexplicable reason that I can't even begin to comprehend, I introduced Cindy as "Beth". Needless to say, she was at the minimum perplexed, and at the maximum... not happy.

On the way home from Manhattan, there are about 20 miles of hills before you get to the flat land that lasts all the way to the Rockies. Of course, there was no cruise control in those days, but I was going a consistent speed down I-70. However, as we went up and down the hills, we would pass a couple semis (tractor trailers) going up and they would pass us going down. After this happened a few times, Cindy started complaining that it was my driving - as if it mattered anyway. No doubt she was embarrassed. Although I liked all the mothers of my girlfriends and wives over the years, I really liked her mom because when we got back to Larned, she explained to Cindy that semis slowed down going up hills and sped up going down and that it wasn't my fault. It's amazing how you remember some things, but forget 99% of the rest.

I actually got my first traffic ticket on that same trip. We were driving on a four lane road with a median. I went through an intersection and looked down the cross roadway and saw some cars had been pulled over. I remember making the boastful and ignorant comment that I would never get a ticket as long as I lived. Within seconds, there was a highway patrolman on my tail with lights flashing. As it turns out, two perpendicular highways met at that intersection and it was a four-way stop. The patrolman couldn't understand how I could not have seen the signs. He indicated there had been several deaths there recently and asked if we would be willing to travel back to the intersection with him and drive through it so he could inquire about what we saw (or didn't see). So, we did. They had big stop signs, but as I recall, I was in the lane next to the median and a semi was ahead of me and to my right side. I think he began slowing for the stop sign, but it was hidden from me until I passed him. By that time, it was out of my peripheral vision. Nowadays, of course, you don't have intersections like that, you have clover leafs - or at the minimum, flashing red lights and a stop sign on the median. BTW: I *was* ticketed! I may be the only person in history to make the boast I would never be ticketed only to be ticketed within minutes.

And, while I'm talking about trips, the next summer we went to Wilson Reservoir which was about an hour north of us. We spent the day there and went out on a boat with some other people. The strange thing about it is that somehow I lost my billfold. I noticed it just as we were getting off the boat and immediately began looking for it. I had it before I got in the boat and I wasn't in the water. Besides, I don't know how it could have come out of my back pocket anyway. I never found it.

As it turns out, it's the only billfold I ever lost, but more interesting than that, it was my first billfold and I only owned three others the rest of my life. My final billfold was one I had from the time I was 37. For years many people tried to buy billfolds for me, but I refused to use them. Consequently, they quit trying. I think I saw it as a symbol of cheapness - which I was/am proud of – all beat up and torn.

COOL FACTOID: Cindy had a 1966 Marlin. Few people today know what that was, but it was made by Rambler. It was yellow with a roof-wide black stripe down the back. What made it cool was that on the dashboard where it had the word "Marlin", she had crossed the "t".

Aw, shucks.

We dated until the beginning of my senior year and her freshman year of college. She went to a JUCO in Great Bend and it was one of the reasons I transferred to Great Bend my senior year. It was a great plan, but I didn't count on her sprouting wings and wanting to fly. It wasn't long before I had lost her to some college guy. It was beyond devastating. The night we broke up, I drove to Larned where my mom worked nights at Larned State Hospital. I hunted her down and I cried my ass off.

The single best thing I ever remember my mom and dad doing for me was they took me to Manhattan, Kansas the next day to see Charles at college. I got to see him and another friend from Larned that was also a year older. That helped immensely. It still took months to get over Cindy and to my last dying breath, she was always special to me.

> "One's first love is always perfect until one meets one's second love."
> -- Elizabeth Aston

My second great love was when I was a sophomore in college. I met an incoming freshman girl named Elaine Kay (Lainie Kay) on the first day of school. It didn't take long before I was crazy in love with her. We dated all through my sophomore year.

The Christmas break was about three weeks long and that was an eternity for me because she went home to Scottsbluff, Nebraska and I stayed and worked in Aggieville. I had a few days off right around Christmas and there were some other kids that I knew who lived a couple hours away - in the direction of Scottsbluff - that were going home for a few days.

Scottsbluff is probably a 6-7 hour drive from Manhattan, Kansas. I had a car, but was too poor to pay for that much gas. Besides, the clunker I had might not make it there and back. So, I took off, riding with my friends early on Sunday, December 23rd. They dropped me off on the edge of their town and I started hitchhiking - something you could still do in 1972.

I got a few more rides and about 9PM on Sunday, I made it to her house. She was shocked to see me, of course, but I got to meet her parents and stayed overnight in the family room. I spent most of the next day (Christmas Eve) with her and her family. Her dad asked me a question... "If John is 14 years older than Mary and John is 56, how old was Mary when John was twice her age?" I don't know why I remember the question except that when I answered "14" in about five seconds, he thought I was a genius. Elaine was a daddy's girl. If he thought I was a genius, then in her eyes, I was.

But, I wasn't part of the family and I had come uninvited and I had to get back to work in Manhattan. So, about 3PM on the 24th, Elaine took me out to the edge of Scottsbluff and we said our good-byes. It took a long time to get halfway across Nebraska. About 10PM, I made it to Grand Island and decided to take a bus. The last one of the night took me to Lincoln - which was about two hours north of Manhattan. By the time I got there, it was 1AM on Christmas Eve.

The bus station was deserted, but I found someone and asked them where the police department was. Fortunately, it was only a couple blocks away. So, I walked over there, asked them what they thought I should do. They said they would drive me to the edge of Lincoln, but that's all they could do. I'm not sure I wanted to be on the edge of Lincoln, Nebraska at 2AM on Christmas Eve, but that's where I found myself.

It was so cold, it was unbelievable - and there weren't any cars driving by - and even if there were, there wasn't any lighting where I was. They wouldn't see me until they had passed me and who is going to stop for some*one* or some*thing* at 2AM on Christmas Eve? I had a sleeping bag, so I just curled up in the ditch half frozen until sunlight.

I got up and started trying to thumb a ride. At least 50 cars went by without stopping. This was Christmas Day! I was shocked nobody would stop and I honestly thought I was going to die. Eventually, a couple in a VW picked me up. They were going to Manhattan and they dropped me off at my house.

Was it worth it? Who knows what I thought at the time? Today... of course not. But, I was 1) 19 years old, 2) an idiot and 3) in love. All three are recipes for disaster. Add them together and you get some kind of harmonic convergence - the perfect storm - a logarithmic explosion of hormones run amok.

One day in the spring, Elaine and I went to Tuttle Creek Reservoir just north of Manhattan for a picnic. We drove her car and parked up on a hill where there were picnic tables. However, we wanted to be closer to the lake, so we walked down to an area just above the water. About 10 minutes later, we heard a bunch of noise – crashing and sticks breaking. I could see through the trees her red Fiat making its way down the hill. At some point I lost sight of it, but I heard a louder bang and then a splash.

We raced over there and sure enough, Elaine's car was floating in the lake. I immediately jumped into the water and grabbed it and tried to drag it to shore before it sank. Almost immediately, there was a boat pushing the car and a few other people were in the water helping me. We got it back to land, but the front quarter panel had been damaged. Still, it eventually drove again.

The mystery was that when the tow company came and hooked it up to a cable and tried to pull it up the hill, the car didn't want to roll. It was only at that time that I unlocked it, got inside and disengaged the parking break so that the tires were free for it to be pulled up the hill. How it rolled down the hill with the parking brake on or what got it started or how it missed all those trees in the first place is a complete unknown - although some other people at the picnic site on top of the hill said they saw kids hanging around it.

I don't really have any better place on this site to mention four-leaf clovers, so I'll tie it into Elaine. For some really strange reason, I've always been obsessive about looking for four-leaf clovers. When we were growing up in Topeka, we lived in a crackerbox house from ages 6-9. In the front yard, there were patches of clover. There must have been some sort of mutation going on because I remember finding tons of four-leaf clovers and many five-leafers, even a six or two. I can't trust my memory, but I think I may have even found a seven-leafer.

Maybe it was that experience which would result in my almost complete inability to walk by a clover patch and not stop and start looking. This stayed with me my entire life. When I used to ride my bike a lot on the trails in Johnson County, I would often stop, get off and start looking for four-leafers. It used to irritate my ex-wife (Teri) because she didn't have any interest except to keep biking.

Whenever I would walk through a park, I would stop and bend down and look. And, trust me, if I only had one talent in the world - it was identifying a four-leaf clover in the middle of a patch.

One summer day after my sophomore year of college, I was working construction and just walking along with another guy. Without breaking stride, I bent down and snagged a four leaf clover and showed it to him. He was absolutely amazed - even dumbfounded. I don't think he ever believed that I had just picked it and hadn't either had it in my hand or planned it before we were started walking.

That previous year when I was dating Elaine, I would go over to her dorm to pick her up. There were clover patches outside the dorm. In those days, you didn't go up to a female's room in a dorm and there were no coed dorms. There was a receptionist of sorts and I would ask her to tell Elaine I was there. While I waited, I would slip out the front door, look through the clover and pick a four-leafer. When she came down, I would hand her a four-leaf clover - kind of my signature way of greeting her. I did that many times and it sort of became a tradition.

Elaine and I dated throughout my sophomore year, but we broke up in the summer. I had driven her home after school to Scottsbluff and then was heading to the other side of Nebraska to Lincoln where I would work that summer. About a couple hours outside of Scottsbluff, I happened to notice a piece of paper on the floor of my car. I reached over and picked it up and it was some hand-written notes by Elaine - sort of a to-do list.

One of the things on the list was to talk to her older sister about me. She indicated she didn't love me and wanted to break up. OMG, I was shell-shocked. I stopped at the next town and got on a pay phone and called her. I asked her about it and she didn't deny it. I never knew if she intentionally left it there for me to find - hoping that would serve as the easy way out. We broke up on the phone. It was just about as hard on me as when Cindy and I broke up two years earlier.

Of course, I loved both of my ex-wives. I still do in a different way. But, the truth is that nobody who came after Cindy and Elaine could match how I felt about them. That's just the way it is when you are young. Everything is either perfect or it's the end of the world. Ultimately, it was both, but I survived as we all do.

My Thoughts

These later essays (including those that follow) give us less insight into Martin's choice of suicide, but each reveals one or two important facts. This essay on his first two loves reveals that Martin was not a complete isolate at high school. He had a good friend, Charles. He also had a girlfriend. He also dated and fell in love at college.

The second interesting detail is that, despite what he said about his cold parents earlier in his essays, when his college girlfriend rejected him, he went home to his mother and cried in her arms. His parents then took him to see his best friend Charles. This indicates that the bond between Martin and his parents was stronger than I thought and that they helped him emotionally when he was in crisis. Perhaps his family was not quite as dysfunctional as he would have us believe?

Chapter 23

Health

One of the major reasons people commit suicide is because of poor health. As I explained in "*Why*" and "*Why Not?*" to the left of this page, health has nothing to do with it for me. I've always thought I had pretty good health. After all, I never drank or smoked and I was within reasonable weight limits for my size. You may have no interest in this, but here is a summary.

I mention this elsewhere, but I didn't miss a scheduled day of work in over 30 years leading up to my death. I don't even know what it means to be too sick to work. I'm thankful to God for having such good fortune and I sympathize with those who don't.

I can only begin to imagine the suffering that some people go through before ultimately deciding to end their life. There are probably millions of elderly people who would choose to end their life if they had the option. Of course, they don't. The family doesn't have an option either unless the person is brain dead. Being brain dead (something I *can* almost identify with) isn't so bad because you don't know the difference. But, it's also no reason to live. Anything less than that means experiencing the suffering – and for what?

No parent should ever see a child die, so if a child is struggling, they try to stay alive as long as they can. Besides, they might live long enough to beat the problem. The reward is a long healthy life and maybe becoming the next President of the United States. Who knows? That all makes sense.

But, when someone has lived their life and the only thing left is suffering, it's time to go! Obviously, I say it's time to go because I say it for myself and I haven't suffered at all.

There are only four times I've been sick in the last 30+ years and three of them were due to my own stupidity - two of which I talk about elsewhere on this site. The fourth was having an appendicitis attack.

One morning in 2002, started feeling pain and sickness around 6AM. By 9AM, I had to go to the emergency walk-in clinic nearby. They diagnosed me with an appendicitis attack and referred me to a local hospital. I was scheduled for 1PM, so I went home and worked on the computer for a couple hours even though it was miserable.

I went to the hospital. In no time they had me under the knife. I had laparoscopic surgery – which means they only make a small incision near the naval and go in from there. Actually, I think they made two or three small incisions, but they only required a couple stitches.

I stayed overnight in the hospital Monday, but went home Tuesday at noon. And, this is a fact… I was singing in choir practice on Wednesday night. So, the point of this is that it's the worst physical problem I ever had and it was no big deal at all.

I also mentioned this event under *Living Donor* to the left.

I bring up the other three times I got sick because you might find it interesting how anyone could be so stupid!

1. The first was on my honeymoon in 1981 with Chris. I have a section to the left called "*Honeymoon…s*" where I tell the story in detail. The short version is that I popped a bunch of Vivarin (200mg caffeine) to stay awake driving to Florida on an empty stomach on my honeymoon night when I should have known better. They made me sick enough that I had to go to the emergency room of a hospital in Tennessee. I was stupid.

2. The second time was also when I was on vacation - this time in Galveston in 1990. I discuss this episode in a section to the left called "Trips and Travel". The short version of this is that I and my wife Chris decided to take a fishing trip out into the Gulf of Mexico. But, I opted for the eight-hour version instead of the four-hour and I picked a day when the wind made the seas rough and I didn't prepare by taking Dramamine or anything else. I was sicker than a dog during the entire voyage. I was stupid.

3. The third time was in 2001. I had given blood at the church and while I was there I stupidly let them give me a shot to prevent the flu - stupid, especially since I never got the flu! Supposedly, these flu shots are incapable of *creating* the flu, but I beg to differ. Early in the afternoon, I went out dirt bike (bicycle) riding where I completely exhausted myself. Yep, I got sick for the next 24 hours. Even *if* the flu shot wasn't responsible – which I maintain it was – I should never have exerted myself like that after giving blood. I was stupid.

Those are the only four times I've been sick in my adult life. The appendicitis attack was relatively small potatoes and the three other times I got sick because of my own stupidity totaled no more than the equivalent of a couple days.

I don't have broken bones or muscle problems or ligament problems or allergies or anything else. I only take acid indigestion pills to keep that under control. The pills do the job. Of course, as I have gotten older, I can't do what I used to. In fact, over the last couple years, I've noticed my ability to run or bike or move furniture to be considerably more difficult in terms of endurance. But, I don't exercise all that much, so I was probably lucky to get as many good years out of my body as I got.

I've never eaten properly. My personality is so obsessive that once I started working on something, I couldn't stand to put it down until I was done. This web-site is a challenge in that respect because it's taken many weeks and I have had to start and stop dozens, if not hundreds, of times.

When I was working in the 1980's I started skipping lunch because it meant taking a break and I didn't want no stinking breaks. I never ate breakfast so it turned into a lifestyle whereby I would eat once a day – supper.

As years and years went by, that became so normal that I never even thought about food before supper. I would eat enough at supper that I wasn't ever hungry any other time. In fact, eventually, I forgot what the feeling of hunger even was. Trust me, when I was a kid I knew. The best meal we would have growing up was macaroni with a can of tomato soup spread over it. YUK!

Still, as I got older, I gained weight. I eventually got up to 190 pounds when ideal weight probably should have been 160. Within months of my suicide I lost 27 pounds and dropped back to a low of 163 in order to donate a kidney. I didn't want them rejecting me because of weight. The way I did it was to simply not eat every third day or so and to give up anything fattening. It only took about four weeks to lose the first 21 pounds. It was unbelievably easy. At one point just before I bottomed out at 163, I only ate seven days out of 17 - one meal each time. As hard as it will be for anyone to believe, I never felt hungry even after four straight non-eating days. I only ate on the fifth day because I was feeling weak and decided I probably better get some energy.

I've always been pretty disciplined with respect to eating. For Lent I would give up Ice Cream, Chocolate and Pizza. That wasn't that hard except for Pizza. I've always said...Four P's to a healthier you – Pizza, Pepsi, Poop and Pee.

So, losing 27 pounds wasn't too tough. The other reason I did it was that I wanted to make sure my blood results were acceptable when donating an organ. Again, I didn't want to be rejected as a donor just because I hadn't been eating right.

Still, I ate *what* I wanted and I only ate one meal a day - and even then, not every day. I'm proof (physically) that you can do that and survive just fine... unless, of course, you *choose not* to survive at the age of 60.

My latest blood results (2012) were all within the acceptable parameters.

	Ideal	Martin (2012)
Cholesterol	100-199	176
Triglycerides	0-149	107
LOL-Cholesterol	0-99	99
HDL-Cholesterol	>39	55
VLDL-Cholesterol	5-40	21
Chol/HDL Ratio	0-5.0	3.2
LDL/HDL Ratio	0-3.6	1.8
Glucose	65-99	91
Hemoglobin	4.8-5.6	5.6

I'm fairly confident these numbers would be even better if I were to have gotten blood results in 2013. But, I knew it didn't matter since I wasn't going to live much longer and since I only cared about being healthy enough to donate an organ.

My Thoughts

The only noteworthy statement here is that Martin says that he can identify with being brain dead! He has senior moments, to be sure, but that is a long way from being brain dead. Cognitive therapists, such as Albert Ellis and Aaron Beck, call this thought pattern *catastrophizing* or *magnification* – seeing an event as much worse than it really is.

Chapter 24

Sleep Deprivation

Needless to say, there are a lot of things about me that are odd. I only eat one meal a day. I work constantly. I've been married twice with no kids. I'm obsessed with numbers. I'm never sick and on and on with my oddities – not the least of which is this site. But, perhaps the strangest thing about me is/are my sleeping habits.

Actually, there probably has never been a more inapt word than "habits". When and how I sleep is anything but habitual. It's like the old discussion about a basketball player that scores 20 points and then 2 and then 25 and then 7 and then 21... etc. "He's inconsistent" said the announcer. "But, at least he's *consistently* inconsistent" said his partner.

That's one thing you can say for me. For my entire life – or at least as long as I can recall, I've been consistently inconsistent with respect to my sleep. If there was one single thing that I could have changed (fixed) in my life, it would have been the ability to go to bed at 10PM and wake up at 6AM every day religiously.

I can only remember as far back as 12 years old when we moved from Topeka to western Kansas. We lived in the sticks about nine miles from the small town where we were bussed to school. We were almost at the end of the bus route. We lived on a corner and the bus would swing by our house and then turn and go half a mile to another house with a long driveway. Then, it would retrace its tracks and come back by our house the second time.

I remember many times – perhaps hundreds – when one of my family would holler that the bus just went by. That would be my wake-up call. I had about four minutes to get up, get ready, get dressed, get my stuff and make it to the corner before the bus would return. And trust, me, I wasn't organized in those days like I am now. I was reinventing the wheel every time I woke up.

The problem was that I wouldn't go to bed until 3AM and the reason why was because my mind was always racing. I was playing some kind of mental sporting event that I made up to keep from going crazy in the middle of nowhere. So, I wouldn't get tired until the middle of the night no matter how little sleep I had the night before.

Of course, for the majority of my adult life, I had to get up and go to work at normal times. I can assure you, I hated it! And, the reason why was because I never got over the desire to stay up as late as humanly possible. I think the reason was because I somehow viewed the end of the day as the end of one of the only days I would ever have in this world.

Even at that age, I was thinking along those lines. I wanted to stretch each day as long as I could and that meant not going to bed.

You can say "Where were your parents?", but my mom worked nights and my dad was asleep long before it ever crossed my mind – at least as a teenager.

During my adult life, I would tend to stay up late and get up as late as possible, but I'm sure I only averaged six hours of sleep for many years. On Saturday's I would try to make up for it, but that doesn't work. For much of my life I went to church on Sunday morning, so I wasn't able to make up for it then anyway. Consequently, I feel like I was sleep-deprived most of my life. I have no idea whether that is part of why I never was able to smell the roses or why I always saw the glass half empty. Maybe it is, maybe it isn't. But, it is what it is, regardless of why.

There were times between businesses that I was involved with where I could experiment with sleeping habits. I tried everything. One that worked for a while was staying up 36 hours and sleeping 12. I felt that was the most efficient because I had more prime hours in which I could work.

I've never awakened feeling fresh. It's just not in the cards. I used to comment that it was 2-3 hours after I got up before I felt 100% awake. Others would tell me they felt 100% awake within 15 minutes or less. I envied that! So, for me, the fewer times I had to get up, the better. In a 48-hour cycle, if I only had to get up once, that was being more efficient. But, that system became impractical and I had to abandon it.

I've experienced a dozen different cycles or systems for sleeping and getting up, but frankly when it's all said and done, going to bed at 6AMish and getting up at 1PMish is just about the best schedule that ever worked for me. Naturally, you can hardly get away with that if you are part of the real world.

When I went to work for the Kansas City Star in 2005, the best thing about the job besides sports statistics was that I went to work at 5PM and got home about 1AM. So, for the last 8+ years, I could go to bed at 6AM and get up at 1PM if I wanted to. I can say without fear of contradiction that it worked better for me than any other cycle – at least any cycle that was consistent with my obligations.

I tried a few other things. I would take sleeping pills in an effort to go to sleep earlier and then take a no doze as soon as I got up, but none of that worked… or if it worked, it didn't work for long.

I'm sure my sleeping habits affected my marriages as you would assume. I'm sure it affected a lot of things in my life. I never sought help for it. I'm not sure whether there is anything anyone could do about it in 2013, much less 30-40 years ago. So I've just lived with it and worked around it.

I'm also sure that I've skipped a night's sleep a few hundred times – similar to skipping eating for a day. I tend to get started doing something and I don't want to stop. If I'm awake and working, I want to continue until I can't. If I'm sleeping, it's pretty much the same thing. Don't change me from the state I'm in!

I've always been like that. I stall taking a shower, but once I get in, I don't want to get out. I stall eating, but once I start, I don't want to stop. I'm just obsessive about disliking change. When I'm traveling by car, I don't want to stop until I almost run out of gas. When I'm working on the computer, I don't want to stop until I look at the clock and realize I only have three minutes to get somewhere I'm supposed to be. Consequently, for my whole life I've run five minutes late.

When I was a freshman in college, the dorm was right across the driveway from the building where I had my first class – at 7:30 AM on MWF. You can imagine that having lived in the middle of nowhere for all my teenage years, by the time I got to college, I was ready to have fun! So, we stayed up well into the night playing cards or whatever. 7:30 AM came *way* too soon.

Well, actually 7:27 came *way* too soon. My roommate had a digital alarm clock. In 1971 that was fancy-smancy. When it clicked over to 7:27, it would hum for about three seconds before it went into alarm mode. I remember hearing that hum and thinking… "Oh, God no!" At 7:27 the alarm went off and by 7:32 (Are you sitting down?), I was in class.

In that class we had the old wood chairs that had the writing surface as part of the chair. I used to go to the back row, tilt it back against the back wall and sleep. One day, the feet of the chair slipped out from under me and I feel back. The chairs had a curved piece of wood to support the back. That piece shattered. Needless to say, it caused a huge commotion and (although I blocked out the consequences), I'm sure I got into some trouble.

That story is a microcosm for my sleep problems. It's had a major effect on my life, although in any given day I wouldn't say it mattered. But, over the course of the last 48 years (at least), it's been as important to the levels of normalcy, sanity and success as anything else – and perhaps *more* than anything else.

Since there wasn't any other logical place to recount my recurring dream on this site, I decided I would do it under this category. For pretty much my entire adult life, I've had a dream every so often that I'm in college and realize all the sudden that I haven't been going to class - that I don't even remember all the classes I signed up for or where they were located. The problem is that it's nearing the last few days of the semester. Naturally, I'm walking all over the place trying to figure out courses, days of the week, room numbers, etc.

It's a pretty frustrating dream as you might imagine. Not life or death, but when you are in college… it seems like it. I decided not all that long ago to Google that dream on line and see if anyone else has ever experienced it. To my amazement, a lot of people have. In fact, shortly thereafter, I mentioned it to a friend (Scott) and he said he had the same recurring dream.

I suspect it is something that is triggered whenever a person is facing a deadline and has some anxiety over it. If that were the case, then I shouldn't have had the dream once since I left the KC Star in February of 2012. However, I have had it a few times since then. Of course, knowing the *ultimate* deadline was coming up August 15, 2013 might have been a trigger for it.

My Thoughts

It is important for Martin to see himself as odd. As he tells about these facets of his life, it does seem as if he is proud of his idiosyncrasies.

His sleeping pattern seems to indicate that he is an evening person, and there is some research evidence (from Chelminski and colleagues, 1999) that evening people are more prone to depression (and attention deficit hyperactivity disorder [ADHD]).

Finally, Martin tells us that he has trouble remembering the first twelve years of his life. My own personal experience suggests that the events when he was twelve (the move to rural

Kansas) were quite traumatic for him and that there may have been crises in the home during those years. My parents separated when I was twelve, and I have very few memories from the first twelve years of my life.

Chapter 25

Living Donor

I don't want this to turn into a rant – and Lord knows I can rant with the best of them… but, it's not going to be especially pretty, that's for sure. I'm not naming any names and I'm not even going to indicate sex. But, I have a story to tell that might help someone in the future.

Late last year (2012) I decided the single most important thing I wanted to do before I turned 60 on August 15th, 2013 when my life was to end was to donate any and all organs that I could possibly donate. So, I began researching it.

I discovered lists on the web of people who were requesting organ donations. I presume these are people that are on some waiting list somewhere, but way down the line. Whether or not they will die before they get an organ, I'm sure some will. I suspect a lot of them will. I thought seriously about contacting one of them by random and going through that process. The other option was going through Midwest Transplant Network (MWTN) here in Kansas City. At least with MWTN, I could be sure that the next available person (whoever that would be) who matched up with me would get the organ and so, ultimately, that's the route I took.

Let's back up about 11 years. I also mention this episode in the category called "*Health*" to the left.

One morning around 6AM in 2002, I started feeling pain in my abdomen. By 9AM, I had to go to the emergency walk-in clinic nearby. They diagnosed me with an appendicitis attack and referred me to a local hospital. I was scheduled for 1PM, so I went home and worked on the computer for a couple hours even though it was miserable. That's how obsessive I am about work. But, I digress.

About noon, I headed over to the hospital. Within a couple hours they had me under the knife. I had laparoscopic surgery – which means they only make a couple small incisions near the naval and go in from there. The incisions only required a couple stitches, which were the only stitches I've had in my entire life.

I stayed overnight in the hospital Monday, but went home Tuesday at noon. And, this is a fact… I was singing in choir practice on Wednesday night. So, the point of this is that it's the worst physical problem I ever had and it was no big deal at all.

Because of the fact that I knew I wasn't going to be alive more than 7-8 more months and because I remembered my only other laparoscopic surgery to be relatively painless, I decided that the gift of life to someone was something I simply could not ignore.

Whether or not my donating a kidney will actually save a life is sort of subjective. At least it's a little subjective if you go through channels and the next person on the list gets the transplant. If that person doesn't get it from you, then they will get it from someone else. So, technically, it probably didn't save *their* life. However, by donating, it moves *everyone* forward one slot. And, that means somewhere down the line, it very likely does save *someone's* life – even if it isn't the person that received your kidney.

Frankly, I didn't care who it was that received the organ and I didn't care if they knew who I was. None of that mattered to me. Consequently, I had no requirements or restrictions about proceeding forward – only that the sooner it was done, the better. My original hope was that it could be done by the end of March.

I've mentioned kidney, but of course, they can also take part of the liver. They can even take one of the two lungs. In all cases, the original donor can continue to live normally. Personally, I would have been happy to have one kidney and part of a liver taken, but MWTN doesn't deal with livers for what reason I don't know.

So, I contacted MWTN in early January to start the process. That was a mistake. In retrospect, I should have either gone to someone that I knew needed it and who had a personal urgency or I should have contacted a transplant hospital directly – such as the University of Kansas Medical Center which likely would have saved some steps of bureaucracy.

I'm writing this so that just in case anyone out there decides to become a living donor, you can learn from my experience. Again, I'm not going to name names because this isn't about anyone's personal accountability. It's about the *system* as much as anything else.

In theory, there would be no problem whatsoever with accomplishing what I wanted to do in the amount of time I planned for it. It could almost certainly have been done in four months or less. I pretty much assumed that to be true from the beginning and it's why I was starting the process in early January.

By now, you have probably figured out that I did not donate a kidney – and for that, I'm deeply sorry. Outside of my two failed marriages that were my fault, it's probably the single most disappointing thing that has ever happened in my life. The difference is that in this case, it was not my fault.

I did everything humanly possible to make this happen short of walking into a transplant surgeon's office, taking out a knife, slicing open my gut, reaching in, yanking out a kidney and slapping it on his desk.

For whatever reason(s) the entire process moved at a snail's pace, even though according to the MWTN web-site (and confirmed by MWTN staff) anyone making an organ donation must be no older than 60. Since my birthday is August 15th and I turn 60, that alone should have moved the process along more quickly.

I started the process with a phone call and then got some literature in the mail. I immediately re-contacted the person and asked about the next step. Anyway, it seemed like each step took much longer than necessary. Even though that's true, I eventually had a meeting with two people at MWTN on February 20th which went very well. The initial meeting was to make sure that I understood what the process of donating really meant, to answer questions, to evaluate my mental well-being, etc. Even though it took a while to get to that meeting stage, it was still six months until my 60th birthday.

One of the things they wanted to be sure about was that I wasn't under some kind of stress in my life such that surgery might create health problems with me – presumably with the heart. And, they also wanted to make sure that I wouldn't be hurt financially and that my family wouldn't be put in a position where they were unable to depend upon me.

I made sure they understood that I lived alone, didn't have financial problems, didn't have an iota of stress in my life because I was retired and that they probably weren't going to find anyone who had less of an issue with those three areas than me.

They had required that I have someone who would be a person that could take care of me after I went home from the hospital if necessary. Like I said before, I had my appendix out on a Tuesday afternoon and I was singing in choir Wednesday night. So, I wasn't concerned about needing anyone's help. Nevertheless, they were adamant about it and so I asked someone to be that person and that person agreed. I didn't tell anyone else about it and would not have told anyone unless I had to.

The reason is obvious. Look at all the time this person has spent in conversations with me about it. If they didn't know about it in the first place, the time would never have been wasted. So, I only discussed it with one person and that person agreed to watch over me after I left the hospital.

As I say, the meeting with MWTN in late February went very well. I enjoyed it and I think they did to. I filled out some paperwork. The one issue that seemed to be problematic was that I did not have health insurance - had not had it since it ran out after I left the Kansas City Star nearly a year earlier. Since I'm never sick and there was nothing wrong with me as far as I was concerned, I had thought I would wait until the national health insurance issue was settled before I decided what to do, but even then I wasn't going be alive beyond August 15, 2013 anyway - so why waste money on health insurance?

To clarify, the insurance company for the person *receiving* the organ covers all costs for the transplant. However, they (MWTN and probably KU Med) want the donor to have insurance as well just in case there are issues that come up later that perhaps are arguably not related to the surgery. In the worst case, the *donor's* insurance would cover it. I get all that and indicated I would obtain insurance the moment I was approved.

The other thing that came up in the meeting was that I would need a blood test to determine lots of things. I had taken blood tests the year before (2012) and I knew I had those results at home. So, when I went home that day after the meeting on February 20th, I immediately emailed them the results. The main thing they were looking at were the results for BUN (14, ideal is 6-24), Creatinine, Serum (.96, ideal is .76-1.27) and BUN/Creatinine Ratio (15, ideal is 9-20). No problems.

In addition, I reiterated in that email on February 20th that I would be willing to get insurance within 24 hours if that is what was required.

They mentioned in the meeting that the longest delay in the process would be getting my situation approved by some "board" that evaluates and approves donors. I also got the impression that it is very unusual, if not rare, for a living person to donate an organ to someone who is not a friend or family member.

This process took forever. I would periodically email them asking what was the latest and so forth. Although I was never critical and I was always polite (unfortunately, not normally my best quality), I made sure to add a sense of urgency to every communication.

I believe this approval "board" meets irregularly, if at all. So, getting to them and getting their approval is a time-consuming process. If a *specific* person's life was on the line, I'm sure it could be done quickly. Apparently because nobody *specifically* was in danger of dying, it drug on and on and on.

Finally, they decided they had enough approvals to move forward. On May 10th, I received this word… "I have everything I need to refer you to a transplant center for their workup!" I was finally scheduled to get a blood test at MWTN on May 22nd - which was just under three months from my birthday.

Since early in 2013 in preparation for this donation, I had lost 25 pounds (peaking at 27) – from 190 to 165 – which is pretty ideal for 5'7" – especially for being 59 years old. I had also been doing more exercising and I had mostly cut out any sweets as the worst numbers for my 2012 blood tests had been related to glucose and cholesterol levels even though they were within the ideal range, just a little high.

I was confident that all of the typical things they look for in blood tests would be way below the high end of ideal. As it turns out from the blood results in late May, two of them (I believe I'm right about that) were slightly above "ideal". There is just no way that's possible in my opinion barring something odd. Even so, I didn't know these results for over a month - late June!

Finally I was contacted by someone from KU Medical Center in *late June*. We discussed the insurance issue and I reiterated I would get insurance the next day once I realized that it was going to happen. This was when I heard that I had a couple things about my blood count that were too high. I explained that I had lost 25 pounds and had been working out and hadn't had much in the way of sweets for months. So, we discussed what could have caused these counts to be high.

Keep in mind that even though a couple things were a little high, they were not saying they wouldn't perform the transplant. In fact, they seemed very interested. The person at KU Med brought up fasting as a potential issue that had to do with the blood count and whether I had been fasting. I'm treading on thin ice here because I'm not a medical doctor – I just play one on TV.

I explained that I eat one meal a day and that's all. However, before I go out in public, I usually have a fruit slush and there is some sugar in it because I also mix a non-diet uncola with the fruit juice, banana and ice. I also swallow about five altoids and stick a couple others in my mouth. I hadn't eaten in roughly 18 hours at the time I got my blood taken. The person seemed to think all of that could have been the reason for a couple high blood counts.

In any event, as I was positive my numbers would be better in 2013 than 2012 – and they were all within the ideal range even in 2012… I was sure that another test (assuming I was told what to do and what *not* to do ahead of time) would yield very good results.

So, the blood test and insurance issues should not have been a problem. On July 2nd, I was called by a second person from KU Medical Center.

Let me back up again.

When I first discussed the hospital with MWTN, there was an opportunity to indicate a preference on which hospital I wanted to go to. I didn't really care except that I believe there were three choices and the other two were on the Missouri side. Since I live in Kansas and since I am a KU fan, I naturally preferred KU Medical Center. I figured even if the doctors couldn't tell a scalpel from a needle, they could at least play basketball for my entertainment. Seriously… I made sure they knew that I just wanted to go to whichever hospital was faster.

In retrospect, I think if I had emphasized KU and stuck with it, it might have helped speed it along. Even more true, if I had bypassed MWTN altogether and simply gone to KU Med, the process would have almost certainly been much faster. The reason I say that is because each hospital has its own waiting list (I believe) and so to determine if there is a match for me, MWTN has to check with all the hospitals and see who has been on the list the longest. I believe it was just coincidence that KU Medical Center was next in line with a match.

When I spoke with the person in late June from KU Med, they indicated the recipient I matched with already had a family member who was going to donate. They also indicated they were not the next in line after that, but were the next in line after that. So, there was another hospital that was next in line, but the person at KU Med did not say which hospital.

Shortly after that I was called by MWTN and asked if I wanted to make KU my sole preference because if I did, then they could skip over the next hospital in line city-wide and go directly to the next person in line at KU Med. The contact at KU had already told me they were interested in me for that person. I stated that I would be happy to make KU Med my only preference if that would speed it up.

I'm writing this on July 2nd. It was just an hour ago (I type pretty fast - almost unbelievably fast, but I've had practice!) that I was called by another person at KU Med that I had not talked to before. They indicated that under normal conditions from the time this phone call would take place to the time of the surgery would probably be at least three months.

Well, I only have month and a half left before I turned 60. That isn't going to cut it. I asked what was involved and was told that I would need a colonoscopy, which I have never had, as well as another blood test, as well as a stress test. It's not that I have a problem with any of those things and am confident they would all have given the green light. The problem was the time frame.

If I knew for a fact that it could be done by August 20th or 25th, I might have seriously considered pushing back my August 15th deathline, but three months from now is October. Besides, I just know – even though the KU people have been very active since I first heard from them and they understand my own personal deadline… I just know that it would drag on. And, even if I was ultimately approved, it would almost certainly be October. Maybe even later.

Anyway, I told the person I would call them the next day (tomorrow) and let them know my decision, but I think I decided within five seconds of hanging up. So, I created this file and started typing.

The fact that I initially contacted MWTN in January and even though it wasn't until February 20th that I had a meeting with them… the fact that it took until June 28th to hear from KU is the problem. That's over four months to simply go from MWTN to KU. It seems inconceivable to me that it could take that long.

The KU people were very apologetic, though I don't know how much of this is their fault. I understand there was a problem in that a person who handled this kind of thing was no longer at KU and the MWTN person didn't know they were gone and so forth. But, my contention is……there was no sense of urgency.

You would think that since this is dealing with people's lives with a life-expectancy clock ticking loudly, "urgency" would be the *one* thing that was, at *all* times, driving the process. When someone walks in offering to donate a kidney when there aren't nearly enough donors for all the people needing organs, the one thing that would happen would be that they put it on fast track to save a life whether the donor was nearing the age deadline or not.

Let me make sure to be clear. I believe that everyone involved and everyone I talked to at MWTN and certainly at KU Med were not only professional and friendly, but probably pretty good at their jobs. I may be wrong, but I think the big problem here was that anonymous living donors are relatively rare and the system just isn't prepared to handle it.

I don't know if my age was something that slowed down the process or the fact that I did not have insurance. I made it clear from the time I was asked that I would get insurance immediately upon knowing if I qualified. I can't do anything about my age, but I was still within their age range, so that shouldn't have been an issue - and they never indicated it was.

For whatever reason February 20th to June 28th seemed to take forever. I hate to put it this way, but some nameless, faceless person out there that needs a kidney is likely going to die because my donation didn't reduce the waiting list by one.

Finally, I want to reiterate how disappointing this is. I'm sick about it. I have spent six months doing everything I can possibly do to save a life. My legacy in life is what it is, but to be able to add saving a life to it would have been an incredible feeling. So, I'm sorry about that and I almost feel guilty for having the August 15th deadline – if for no other reason than I might have been able to be approved and donate a kidney by October or some future date.

But, the fact is that the date is set in stone because I will not be around after August 15th. I made a decision. I will often take a little more time than someone else to make a decision because I'm extremely analytical and I want to weigh all the options. Besides, I'm not impulsive and I hate making wrong decisions. So, when I decided my 60th birthday was the deadline – which was also consistent with the maximum age for a donor, I never reconsidered it and made my plans accordingly.

I'm going out and getting a gallon of chocolate swirl ice cream and eating myself into oblivion!

EDIT: On July 3rd, I called KU Med back and indicated that if it took at least three months from this date, I could not donate the kidney and the reason was because my deadline of August 15th was due to the fact that I would not be around after that. They almost certainly assumed I meant I was moving... but I literally meant "I would not be around."

EDIT: On July 22nd, I heard from one of the people at Midwest Transplant Networks who was very apologetic, but indicated this process could take "6-12" months. For one thing, nobody ever told me "6-12" months until *that very moment*. Secondly, that isn't a *justification* for the snail's pace, but rather an *indictment*. If someone wants to donate a kidney to save a life and the process takes 6-12 months, whether they are told that or not, something is broken. It should be able to be done in 1-2 months in my somewhat uneducated opinion. There are a hundred things that could happen in 6-12 months that could ultimately cause the person to not be able to follow through on a donation - not the least of which is their own death.

EDIT: On July 23rd, I called one of the individuals at KU Med and indicated that I had put together some thoughts about the process and that IMO, it needed to be fixed. I sent this write-up to them - obviously, without any references to August 15th being the end of my life.

EDIT: On August 1st, I got the idea of putting into place a plan whereby the moment I die a number of things would happen. So, I intend to send emails to everyone involved on the 14th of August telling them I have something urgent to say on the morning of August 15th. It took a great deal of work via trial and error, but I figured out how to send delay emails via Google Mail.

Within minutes of the time I expect to end my life, I plan on emails arriving at all of these people's computers telling them what I did, where my body is and begging them to harvest my organs since they have the information they needed. Keep in mind, the issues related to colonoscopy or blood levels or stress tests are for *MY* benefit - to make sure I'm healthy enough to endure the surgery. Once I'm dead, who cares? I've researched the amount of time that specific organs will stay healthy for donation after death and there should be plenty of time to make it happen. In my suicide letter that I am leaving with my body - which is on the property of the Overland Park police station and barely a block from St. Luke's Medical Center, I also beg them to contact the people involved at MWTN and KU Med and to be as cooperative as humanly possible so that my organs could be donated to save one or more lives.

I've left my sister in Topeka in charge of dealing with the relatively few remaining issues after my death. Obviously, I'm not going to tell her that I plan to commit suicide and I wasn't even going to tell her about my failed attempt at a donation. But, then I decided her knowing this story would mean it would be fresh on her mind. When she gets my email just after 5AM on August 15th - the time of my death if everything went right - I will emphasize how urgent it is that she contact the people at MWTN and KU Med and that she put pressure on the police to avoid any delays.

Maybe by some miracle what I was unable to accomplish in *life*, I might be able to accomplish in *death*. And, if this plan fails, I hope someone will get to the bottom of it to find out why. And, if the reason is because of more bureaucracy or red tape or foot dragging or whatever, I hope the process gets scrutinized such that it won't happen with the next Martin Manley.

My Thoughts

Donating organs while living to complete strangers is unusual. Typically, people do this for family members or friends. I have heard of a coach donating a kidney to one of the kids whom he coached. Clearly, doing this came to be very important for Martin – this last altruistic act before his death.

Interestingly, many years ago, Paul Blachly (1971) noted that people who donated blood or organs while alive experienced a satisfying sense of well-being afterwards and had more satisfying interpersonal relationships with others. Blachly thought that this kind of altruistic donation was similar to a sacrifice and that sacrifice might be a useful adjunct to psychotherapy. Going even further, Blachly suggested that this *partial sacrifice* might substitute for *total sacrifice* (suicide), especially for individuals who are anomic and egoistic (that is, alienated or disengaged from society's social ties and social values). Martin wanted desperately to donate a kidney. If this had happened, might his thoughts about suicide changed afterwards? Probably not, but it is an interesting possibility.

Chapter 26

Food and Drink

I'll accept that nobody cares about this category – what foods or drinks I liked. But, it's also true that 1) this is my site, 2) it's my last time to have the podium and 3) food and drink were a big deal to me just like they are to you or anyone else.

I've mentioned on this site that my mom was a miserable cook. I loved her, of course, but please. I can remember a meal we probably had three times a week – macaroni with a can of tomato soup poured over it. Ugh.

Until I left home after high school, I really never knew what it was to eat good – and by that I don't mean expensively, I just mean good tasting, much less filling.

In fairness to my mom, she worked all the time and we didn't have much money. I just don't know how my dad could stand it. At least kids are resilient. Besides, we didn't really know the difference.

Obviously, when I could afford to eat whatever I wanted, I often would. Even so, I was always cheap. I didn't want to spend money on things that would cost very much, so I had to learn how to either accept food that wasn't as good or figure out how to get a great meal for not much money.

From the time I moved back to Topeka in 1978, I fell in love with Godfather's Pizza. I guess they have 622 locations in 39 states, but it's headquartered in Omaha, Nebraska – so it's not surprising there are lots locations in these parts (Kansas City).

My ideal food is pizza and my ideal pizza is a Godfather's All-Meat (no sausage, no Italian sausage - yuk!), extra cheese. That's heaven on Earth right there.

The World is your Oyster." The problem is, I hate Oysters – and I hate Shakespeare! Now, if he had written "The World is your Godfather's Pizza" I might still be around reading him!

After my second divorce in 2004, I started a mission to learn how to have great meals that were cheap and quick – meals I could make myself. I was successful as far as I'm concerned. I've never eaten so good as I have the last nine years even though my budget is $6/day.

Of course, when I eat out – and I do now and then – I pay considerably more than that (duh). But, with respect to the meals at home, it's an average of $6/day and there is no reason it needs to be more than that.

I've mentioned elsewhere that I only eat one meal a day and have for decades. That's supper. So, the entire $6 goes into one meal. It's probably unrealistic to think it could be done if I were eating multiple meals a day, but I see no reason to do that. It takes too much time and probably would cost more.

I became a "one-mealer" in the 1980's and have never looked back. I estimate that the entire amount of time per day I spend buying groceries, preparing my one meal and eating it is less than 30 minutes. I'm all about time efficiency and reducing time spent anywhere I can. That enables me more time to do those things I want to do... like write and crunch numbers.

As much as I loved Godfather's pizza, I simply couldn't justify it because it was so expensive. Most pizza places have really cheap pizzas that you can get for a nickel and a dime, but almost all of them are crap compared to GF. Having said that, even crap pizza is a lot better than most things. Still, I always yearn for GFs.

I finally figured the best way to do it was to order and pick up the jumbo. There is a long-standing $4.00-off coupon on their site for a jumbo and so applying that with tax, it's just over $28. It wouldn't seem like someone as cheap as me could justify a $28 pizza, but here is how it works.

They cut it into 12 pieces. And, unlike most of these other pizza places, including the worst of all – Pizza Hut, the gunk on a GF pizza goes all the way to the edge of the crust. With Pizza Hut, the outside two inches has almost nothing on it. I can't even comprehend how Pizza Hut is still in business. GF is filling, to put it mildly, even for someone like me who can eat a ton.

I'd been losing weight over the past few months leading up to August 15th, but I could still do the GF jumbo thing. I would have three slices each day for four days. That's $7 per day, but I get back to the *average* of $6 because almost every other meal is less than $6.

I love spaghetti, stew, taquitos smothered in cheddar cheese, chef salad, meat loaf, tacos and many other things. I don't snack so that saves money. I buy all my food from Wal-Mart, so that saves money as well.

As to drinks, I remember when I was young, we had little to drink other than water. My dad hated milk, so I decided I didn't like it either. It wasn't until high school that I started making Kool-Aid. I would put so much sugar in it, it was ridiculous. The idea of drinking pop was inconceivable. We couldn't afford a luxury like that.

It probably wasn't until I was in my mid 20's that I started drinking soda. Sometime shortly after that, it became the only thing I drank. No milk, no juices, no tea, no coffee, no beer, no water, no nothing except pop. For many years, I drank Pepsi exclusively. I finally decided I should try to learn to drink Diet Pepsi considering how much I drank. It didn't take long before I had retrained my taste buds into believing it was just as sweet as Pepsi. So, for many years, that's all I drank. Over the last 15 years, I've switched to Sam's Club diet cola for about half my drinks and Sam's Club (non-diet) uncola called Twist Up. A two-liter bottle of each is about 60 cents - less than a far smaller bottle of water. WOW, what a scam those water producers have got going on and what suckers people are that buy it, but I digress.

The other day I was in a fancy Fed Ex retail store where they do everything. I've used them for a number of different jobs for this site. They have candy and cola for sale. There is a little fridge there with several different kinds of pop. They are all the same size - 20 fluid ounces - although they didn't look like they were any bigger than a can of soda (12 ounces). But, let's say 20. The cost was $1.50 each. That's 7.5 cents per ounce.

A two-liter bottle of Sam's cola or a variety of other soft drinks is about 60 cents at Wal Mart. A two-liter bottle has 68 fluid ounces. So, that means it's less than a penny per ounce. And, that means that the pop I drink at home is about 8-9 times cheaper per ounce than at the

Fed Ex store! This is a classic example of the difference between me (cheap) and someone else who just spends what they have. I would never in a hundred years buy one of those bottles of water for $1.50. And, because of that miserly mentality, I'm able to give away money to quite a few people before I die.

As much pop as I drink, the cost would be prohibitive if I were to pay the rate many people pay. Also, drinking a lot of fluids - whether pop or not is part of why I've always been healthy, but I'll leave that up to the nutritionists to debate.

I drink the diet cola exclusively when I eat. I drink the uncola at other times. Neither seems appealing to me if I were to switch their roles.

About six years ago or so, I decided I wanted to try to figure out how to make a really great fruit slush. I succeeded. This is the best in the world.

First, go to WalMart. Buy a gallon of Robert's Fruit Punch or Robert's Strawberry Banana. Either way works fine. After the first time, you will have an extra empty gallon around. Pour half the fruit juice into each gallon and fill the rest of it with Twist Up.

Take half an unfrozen banana and half a frozen banana. This requires having frozen bananas. To make this work out you have a baggie in the freezer and the bananas inside of it are pre-peeled and cut into fourths.

Then, you take a tray of ice, put it in a blender with two fourths of a frozen banana, one half an unfrozen banana and you fill the blender to whatever approximately 20 ounces would be of the fruit juice. Blend it on high speed and what comes out is heaven. I have one every *morning* (whenever that is).

Obviously, my obsession with eating cheap and only eating one meal a day and only drinking a couple different products is consistent with my overall abnormal and obsessive personality.

By the way, you can check out my cook book – due out in 2014.

My Thoughts

His eating pattern is odd and, again, he seems to be proud of it. His cheapness, of which he also seems to be proud, has enabled him to save money which he can now give to others altruistically.

Chapter 27

Kansas City Star

I spent most of my adult life working for myself or with partners, but after we sold off what we had left, I opted to work for the Kansas City Star. My job was in dealing with sports statistics. Having written three books on sports stats and numerous articles, it was a natural fit for what I figured would be the last 10 years of my life. I didn't quite make it. I left the Star after seven years and left the world after nine. But... close enough.

I abruptly walked away from The Star in early 2012. When I did, there was a lot of speculation as to what happened. I set the record straight over a year ago on my sports blog *SportsInReview.com*. But, for *this* record, I want to reiterate a few things. Besides, a year ago in my SIR post, I did not include anything from the letter of recommendation that I received from the paper's Editor - Mike Fanin.

My last day of work at The Star was February 6th of 2012. I wrote my last article on my blog, Upon Further Review, later that night (early morning) and I began it with…

> "After 3.3 years, almost 2,000 articles and at least one story every day for 653 days in a row, this *may* be my last post on UFR. If so, you'll hear from me in the future and I'll be happy to spell it out…"

I survived approximately nine lay-offs at The Star because I was a workaholic. I never missed a day of work in all the years I was with the company. I rarely even took my vacation. I got 24 days a year and in the last two years, I took seven of 48 days. Company policy was not to pay for days not taken which I fully understood, so I just lost 41 days. I never took breaks, never stopped to eat during a shift, worked my butt off pretty much every minute I was there because… I just wanted to work.

And, that's not all. I was solely responsible for Upon Further Review (the name of the blog at that time). I posted an average of 1.5 stories per day. Every single one of them conceived of, researched by, written by, edited by and posted by … me. I didn't ask for, nor did I receive, help. In fact, I posted at least one story for 653 consecutive days from late April, 2010 until February 6, 2012 and almost every single day before that - despite working full time.

Almost all the work on the blog was from midnight to 6AM after my shift at work. And, on my two days off a week, I worked numerous hours on the blog. Basically, I lived, ate, drank and slept (when I had time) Kansas City sports, Kansas City Star and Upon Further Review. What life?

At The Star, I was the statistics editor which meant I was responsible primarily for the data page(s). When I took it over, it was a cluttered mess IMO. I made every single page organized, cut out widows, aligned the categories, added original content, etc. That took motivation because nobody told, nor expected, me to go that far. I unilaterally made it my mission to enhance and improve the data page(s) because anything I do will be done to the highest level or I'm not going to have anything to do with it. Of course, that commitment took more time and effort and energy. I claimed there wasn't a better data page anywhere in the United States – and I even offered $100 to anyone who could find one. Nobody ever did.

Considering the volume of work I provided and the quality level of that work, I don't know of any time I was ever at risk for losing my job. My performance ratings were always good. But, over time, the job(s) got harder and harder and harder. Why? Simple… nine layoffs.

The amount of work I (alone) was responsible for just kept increasing and increasing. I could only work 70 hours a week for so long before I just couldn't take another second of it… literally. My *last* second was February 6th around 11:55 PM. I wrote my *final article* on UFR that night.

Later, after my blog post and before I left work at 6AM, I wrote a five-page letter to the sports editor outlining my concerns. The rest is more or less history. I never worked another minute for The Star and *officially* ended my employment with the company on Friday, February 24th after a meeting with Mike Fannin, the editor of the paper. I believe we separated on good terms. From his letter of recommendation...

…"Martin's primary role was to produce the Daily Data page, where he was a master at creating clean, organized and unique statistical information. In addition, Martin was instrumental in Upon Further Review, a Kansas City Star-produced sports blog. He served as a valuable contributor to this blog for over three years. Martin was reliable, hard-working and conscientious, and his contributions were highly valued."

And, from the Sports Editor who followed Mike Fannin - Holly Lawton when she left The Star......"Thanks so much for your tremendous work ethic and your perfectionism. I've always valued your contributions, but also you as a person."

Anyway, that's exactly what happened. Every word above is 100% factual.

But, I don't want to leave you with the wrong impression. For all but the final six months – when I felt my personal situation was becoming untenable - I loved the job I had. And, I was able to conjure up the energy required to essentially do *two* jobs. Let's face it, any job that is about sports and stats… I mean come on. What's not to love? So, although the last (roughly) six months were increasingly more difficult and stressful, I have good memories of my years at The Star.

COOL FACTOID PART I: Let's pretend there were no pictures or ads in a newspaper and that it was 40 pages long and had been 40 pages for a 100 years. I estimate there would be roughly 9,000 words per page or 360,000 per day. In 100 years, that amounts to 36,500 days and 13.14 billion words.

COOL FACTOID PART II: On the other hand, my latest $300 home computer has a hard drive of 1TB – one terabyte. That's 1 trillion bytes (or 500 billion letters). If the average word has 6.6 letters plus a space, that means my home computer can hold 65.8 billion words.

COOL FACTOID PART III: The bottom line is my home computer (smaller than a briefcase) can hold every single word ever written in five newspapers for 100 years assuming they are 40 pages every day and no ads. And, if that doesn't explain why the newspaper industry is dying, nothing does.

The Daily Miracle

It never ceased to amaze me how every single day at The Star we would come into work late in the afternoon with nothing, and by midnight we would have this multi-colored many-paged mini-magazine. A few hours later, everyone in Kansas City that wanted it would have it at their door. Lots of stories, data, information – all of it checked and double-checked and as timely as our deadlines would allow.

The Kansas City Star sports department received many awards. I'm not sure there is another paper in the nation that got as many awards per subscriber as ours – including the coveted APSE Triple Crown award on several occasions while I was there. I thought the name of the paper should be changed to "The Daily Miracle" because honestly that's how I viewed it.

Criticisms and the Future of Newspapers

Most of the criticism of The Star sports department was unjustified IMO – at least as it pertains to content. People criticized the paper for being biased toward this or that university... or this or that sport. That was the most common complaint I heard. But they don't have a clue about how much effort went into trying to keep it fair and balanced. Did we make mistakes occasionally? Are we human?

Criticism of newspapers *in general* is a different issue, however. The industry is in major trouble as everyone on earth knows. It's hard to justify to anyone who is computer savvy why they should wait to get the news and sports a day late by going out to their driveway regardless of the weather with no ability to interact with the story and with limitations on the length and content of the story because of space issues. It's seemingly archaic in a digital world.

I honestly believe that in another 20 years, kids will be saying to their parents or grandparents... "You mean you used to have to wait until the next day to get all that information and you couldn't interact with it and you had to go out in the snow or rain and wring out a piece of paper?" It will be very similar to what some of us said to *our* parents or grandparents... "You mean you used to have to go outside in the middle of the night in the rain or snow just to take a pee or poop?" What's the business model for outhouses and corncobs today?

Although that's almost certainly a fair analogy IMO, I will concede that it overlooks one thing. The Star and all newspapers are becoming more and more focused upon analysis as opposed to breaking news. The Star owns KansasCity.com where breaking news takes place.

KansasCity.com is specifically for many of us that get our KC time-sensitive information. The newspaper is for everyone else. And, the one thing newspapers have is quality researchers… with time - *limited* time yes, but more than the time granted to people on line!

Time is a marvelous thing when your mission is… objectivity and accuracy. No matter what happens to The Star in the future, I think it is fairly safe to say *getting it right* will never be intentionally compromised because if it is, there isn't anything else for a newspaper to hang its hat upon.

I'll never suggest to someone that reads The Star… to give it up, but Father Time *is* relentlessly making the argument in place of me or anyone else saying it. The problem is an aging population that has never known anything other than a newspaper is… aging. And, it's being replaced by generations of people that simply will not wait for information under *any* conditions – even if it means greater accuracy. Presumably, the masses figure accuracy will work itself out. If not within the first hour or two, then maybe 12-24. Clearly, that's an unfortunate by-product of a digital world. But, what are you going to do? You can't put the toothpaste back in the tube and everything is about speed and instantaneous delivery. Even Sports In Review had to buck that trend.

Unfortunately, advertisers know the demographics of newspaper readers and they also know people's prime spending ages are when they are in their 30's and 40's. That's the vertical revenue mountain newspapers have to climb, and that's why the large number of layoffs industry-wide. Nothing I (or anyone else) says or does will change the inevitable societal evolution of how information is transmitted – whatever that ultimately becomes. Newspapers and employees of newspapers are just along for the ride.

The People at the Star

I want to take one last opportunity to express my well wishes to everyone at The Star. The editor of the paper (Mike Fannin) is absolutely first rate – a real professional – a super good guy. Opinions vary, but that's mine. Mike was the sports editor for years while I was there before he was promoted. The sports editor today is Jeff Rosen. Jeff is a great guy IMO as well. I wish both of them the best of luck.

The rest of the people that made up the sports desk were/are *very* talented, hard-working people. Having sat among them for as long as I did, I came to appreciate what it takes to create something from nothing, to get it right 99.9% of the time, to make it aesthetically pleasing, to be even-handed, to reach out to as many disparate groups as possible… and to do it *every single day*. Day after day, week after week, month after month, year after year. I believe the paper hasn't missed a printing in over 100 years.

My Thoughts

Martin has not told us yet what were the businesses that he worked for before working for the newspaper. How enjoyable was that work and how much income and savings did they generate?

His description of his working life resembles the description of his eating habits which he himself described as obsessive. The growing stress he experienced working at the newspaper led him to quit, but we have no idea the extent to which, at age 60, Martin could live comfortably in retirement. Has he saved enough in retirement accounts, or is he facing living only on social security?

Chapter 28

Tornado at the Woodlands

On May 4, 2003 my family and I went to the Woodlands (Kansas City, Kansas) for the first (and only) time to watch the dog races. I knew nothing about the sport then and I know nothing about it now – only that a bunch of dogs run around a track at blinding speeds. It's not very entertaining because it's over in just a matter of seconds. No time to build drama or root for one dog to overcome another...

My brother and sister were in town visiting and we had gone to the Royals game the night before. Keep in mind, this was early in 2003. That was the year in which the Royals came out of the gate like gangbusters and were leading the division. However, after a 16-3 start, they were 2-5 over the most recent week. Even so, you can't go wrong with nice weather on Friday night game at the K – though they lost 6-1.

Rather than take in a second Royals game the following day, we decided to go to see the dogs. We had no expectation of anything other than an interesting experience since none of us had ever seen dogs race. After about seven events (approximately half the card) the clouds started getting nasty looking. They suspended the races and indicated tornado watches had been issued. Shortly after that, they announced a funnel cloud had been seen a couple miles SW of the Kansas Speedway. That means it was around five miles SW of the Woodlands. Anybody who knows anything about tornadoes knows they move from SW to NE the vast majority of the time. And, that meant trouble.

So, they told everyone to get away from the windows and to get to the center of the building. Needless to say, about 20 of us men totally disregarded that announcement and immediately went outside to see what we could see. Over the next few minutes, most returned inside as the wind was picking up and there were a few drops of rain. I had my camera and began taking pictures.

[I could] see the beginnings of a tornado dropping out of the sky. By this time, it was past Kansas Speedway and Cabela's - just crossing 435 – roughly two miles from the Woodlands. At that point, I was the only one in the parking lot. I ran back inside to make sure everyone realized we had a tornado that could be a threat. When I turned around to go back outside, one of the officials at the Woodlands tried to stop me. "You can't go out there", he said. I replied with the only thing that came to me … "I'm a professional photographer and this is my job." Of course, I just had this little 35mm camera and barely even knew how to push the click button… and he probably knew it. But, whether he did or not, he said "If you go back out there, you aren't going to get back in because we are going to lock the doors."

Ok, I knew immediately, that was a bunch of crap. I can see it now - some customer banging on the glass doors with a tornado bearing down on him while his family watches in horror… and you won't let him back in? Sure.

But, I didn't care what he said. This was just too exciting. I ran back out to the parking lot and began taking pictures. It was immediately apparent to me that it would miss the parking lot to the south and travel by us on the east, so I knew I was safe.

By the time I took my last picture and the hail started, I was all done with my experience and had the pictures to prove it. As I started back to the huddled masses, a few of them came out to watch the tornado head on toward the Missouri river and beyond.

Most of the people there thought I was insane. Of course, they are right (duh), but it is a badge of honor I wear proudly. If insane means abnormal, count me in!

They cancelled the rest of the races and everyone left shortly thereafter. We viewed a little bit of the damage, but the police had the area cordoned off almost immediately. So, we drove back home to south Johnson County, Kansas.

No sooner had we arrived home than an incredible rainbow arched across the sky. I took a picture of it with the two girls that went with us – Jaime (left) and Marissa.

It's an amazing thing to watch the power and the splendor of weather – from the good to the bad and back full circle in such a short period of time. That was my second biggest thrill at an athletic event, but one I hope doesn't reoccur (#1 was game six of the 1985 World Series).

Ever since I experienced that tornado, I have wondered why it is that sporting events don't seem to get hit by tornadoes. I understand that some are cancelled based on the possibility of storms, but relatively few.

Only one professional baseball game has ever been cancelled to my knowledge because a tornado might form and attack the stadium. That was in early June, 2013 in St. Louis. It just seems like the day will come when there will be thousands of people clustered together for some sports activity and a tornado will come out of nowhere and there will be nowhere to hide.

It didn't happen to the few hundred of us at the Woodlands on May 4, 2003 and it hasn't happened to any others that I know of. Inevitably, it *will* happen someday with hundreds or thousands being injured or killed.

Here is to hoping Mother Nature remains one of those fans that does *not* storm the field!

My Thoughts

We learn that he was on good terms with his brother and sister. They visited, and probably he visited them with his wives. And again, Martin is proud of his "insane" behavior during the tornado when he went outside to photograph it.

Chapter 29

Synesthesia

I very recently discovered that I have an affliction called grapheme-color synesthesia, however I'm not sure I would consider it an *affliction* since the word "affliction" has negative connotations and I don't see it as negative. Grapheme means "letter or number". The synesthesia is the unconscious act of associating two things that most of us would typically see as completely independent of each other - for example tasting letters or seeing sounds.

Most people don't make the connections I make - that being associating colors with a numbers. For most everyone, a three is a 3. Nothing more, nothing less. However, that's not true for me… a three is yellow (duh). I can't remember a time when I did *not* see numbers as colors and it wasn't until the past few years that I actually realized that nobody else I knew saw it that way.

I wonder how it could have taken me so long to realize that I was making a connection that didn't logically exist – and thus, why should it be true for anyone – including me? Nevertheless, at some point, the light bulb clicked on and I decided I wanted to see who else might have grapheme-color synesthesia. The only problem was that I didn't know there was a name for it.

Recently, I sent out an email on the Triple Nine Society message board inquiring about this and one person sent back a response that introduced me to the scientific name for it. Once I had that, I read quite a bit about it – all very fascinating.

It seems that people with synesthesia are pretty much born that way and it is also true that they don't change much over time. In other words, if I see the number nine as brown, I'm going to see it as brown ten years later. If I see the letter Z as black, that's not going to change either.

Many people with synesthesia will use the relationship between colors and numbers or colors and letters to help them remember names or strings of digits. Apparently, this phenomenon has been known about for quite a while, so research is becoming more advanced.

I don't know that it is an indicator of anything about the person – whether related to intelligence or memory, but they have determined the parts of the brain that are responsible for it. Grapheme-color synesthetes tend to have an increased thickness, volume, and surface area of the fusiform gyrus. And, that's about as technical as I care to get with it.

I asked a dozen friends to associate the ten digits 0, 1, 2, 3, 4, 5, 6, 7, 8, 9 with nine colors (alphabetical): Black, Blue, Brown, Green, Orange, Purple, Red, White, Yellow – leaving one digit blank.

To my utter surprise, not only did they not agree at all, but there was hardly any consensus about any pair. They didn't even agree with me. Their results were pure random guesses from what I could see. I found myself looking at their pairs and saying to myself… "wrong, wrong, wrong, wrong, right, wrong, wrong, wrong, wrong" – as though I were grading a test with absolute correct or incorrect answers.

The only explanation for why I would tend to view their responses in such an absolute way is because I see the associations between the numbers and colors as clearly as I see almost anything else. There is very little subjectivity to it from my perspective.

Here are my associations for the nine colors and ten digits. Also shown is my confidence level for each. Most are crystal clear, but not all.

Number	Color	Confidence level
0	Black	100%
1	White	100%
2	Purple	40%
3	Yellow	100%
4	Blue	80%
5	Red	100%
6	Green	100%
7	Orange	100%
---8	Blue	20%
---8	Purple	40%
9	Brown	100%

As you can see seven of the nine numbers are 100% associated with a color. The problem comes with Blue and Purple. Blue could be either four or eight – though I'm more comfortable with it being four. Purple could be either two or eight. Both seem about equal to me.

If I had thought about it, I would have added a 10th color (gray) which would have been a no-brainer at #2 - especially with 0 (black) and 1 (white) and which would then force purple to be #8 and blue #4. Even though the #2 as gray is extremely logical, it doesn't jump out at me for some reason. Maybe too much gray matter or too little gray matter. That, of course, is an attempt at a joke!

Looking only at those seven colors that I am 100% confident of, here are the total number of people who agreed with me out of the 12 that I "tested".

As I said, that's really no more than random agreement. My sister agreed with me on three of them – more than anyone else, but that's probably just coincidence.

The really strange thing about this to me is that, although I can accept (begrudgingly) a person not agreeing on Yellow, Red, Green, Orange or Brown, I'm flabbergasted that anyone would not have 0 as Black and 1 as White. I would think that would almost be *learned*. Computer code is simply 0's and 1's. What two colors go together in a pair more than black and white? And, what two numbers go together in a pair more than zero and one? It just seems obvious. But, none of the other 12 that I "tested" had both a zero as black and a one as white.

Number	Color	Number agreeing
0	Black	1
1	White	2
3	Yellow	2
5	Red	0
6	Green	1
7	Orange	2
9	Brown	3

Considering none of the people I queried seem to have grapheme-color synesthesia, I simply chalked up their "wrongness" to that fact. However, in researching this, it's apparently true the associations made between numbers and colors are almost random among those *with* the affliction. In other words, few people are going to agree with each other even if they are completely confident of what the associations should be based upon seeing them in their mind.

As to alphabetical associations with color, that isn't something I can identify with at all. That just seems weird and I want to say "Those people are just weirdoes.", but ... Although I write prodigiously, I'm overwhelmingly more of a numbers guy. It would probably be an interesting mini-study to determine if those with only *number*/color convictions are "numbers" people while those with only *alphabet*/color convictions are "words" people.

In any event, I don't think the fact that I see numbers as colors has either enhanced or discouraged my ability to deal with numbers. I mostly just see it as an interesting subject.

My Thoughts

The synesthesia is yet another trait that sets Martin apart from others. So much of his life makes him unique in his self-perception.

Chapter 30

Legal

I've never been arrested, much less been in jail. Come to think of it, other than traffic court, I've never been inside a courtroom during a live session. Does that mean I've been perfect all my life? No, but then a foul isn't really a foul unless the referee calls it either.

Actually, in retrospect, I have been in court two times. Both divorces. However, in both cases we separated amicably and either used the same lawyer or no lawyer. But, both cases required appearing before a judge to state that we were satisfied with the terms we had settled upon.

I've tried to abide by the laws of the land. After all, if I didn't, then why should I expect anyone else to. The only exceptions were driving over the speed limit. But, even then, I tried to keep it to seven or fewer miles per hour above the limit on the highway and four or fewer above the limit in town. I figured I would never get a ticket at those speeds and I always felt safe.

The only time I ever had to talk to a policeman when I might be in some kind of trouble was when I was 11 and living in Topeka. I used to swipe a few bucks from my mom's purse and dole them out to kids in my class. I guess I was trying to buy popularity. Who knows? At 11 in those days, kids were far less mature than 11 today, and I was less than average.

My mom figured out it must be happening. We were so poor that $2 was noticeable. She confronted me with it along with my dad and his belt. I was scared of all three! Apparently, one of the kids ratted me out to his dad and he contacted mine. So, I got punished and never did it again.

Part of my punishment was to get a lecture from a policeman. I don't remember much about it except that my dad worked at the Topeka Public Library. He majored in history and read constantly. So, it was an ideal place to work even if it didn't pay much. I remember sitting in a car with a policeman and my dad in the parking lot of the library. I don't know what he said, only that I'm sure I felt like I just committed murder or something. It was easy to intimidate 11-year olds in those days.

That's my big run-in with the law.

Of course, I've gotten driving tickets - one of which was in Great Bend, Kansas. I was anal even as a senior in high school. So, when I got the ticket, I noticed there were a bunch of discrepancies. I believe there were four. He noted the wrong intersection – off by a block. It was just after midnight and he wrote the previous date on it. He spelled my name wrong. And, one other discrepancy which I forget. So, I went to traffic court and told the judge I was contesting it because whoever this person was, it wasn't me. That wasn't my name and I wasn't even in Great Bend on the date shown – much less at that intersection. Anyway, the judge rolled his eyes and said… "Pay the fine… next case."

I had seven tickets by the time I was 30. None of them were for anything serious, but seven is a fair number. One of them was for rear-ending another car stopped at a light. I was eating pizza and reading the newspaper when it happened, so of course the car in front of me came out of nowhere. How could that be my fault. Just kidding. I vowed never to read the paper and eat pizza at the same time while driving – though I never said anything about one or the other.

As I got older, like most drivers, I sort of forgot where the fire was and slowed down. Interestingly, I've been pulled over for some kind of violation eight times in the past 11 years, but only one of the eight was I given a ticket. Four of them were when I worked at the Kansas City Star and would come home about 1AM or later. Cops were always looking for any excuse to pull someone over so they could nail them on a DUI. Once they figured out that I was just a guy coming home from work that didn't put on his blinker (because there were no cars within a mile), he would send me on my way. I've never drank, so that wasn't an issue with me.

COOL FACTOID: Amazingly, I was never drunk a single time in my life. I thought about getting drunk in early August, 2013, just to see what it was like, but decided I would rather have this cool factoid.

> "I hate to advocate drugs, alcohol, violence, or insanity to anyone, but they've always worked for me."
> -- Hunter S. Thompson

The other three times I didn't get a ticket all happened when I drove to El Paso and back. I got pulled over in Oklahoma on the way down, while in El Paso and then in Kansas on the way back. I was doing something wrong in every case, but they let me off. It must have been the innocent look I gave them.

I got a ticket once in Topeka when I was in my 30's. I won't bother with the details, but trust me it was a situation where 90% of the cars that turned where I turned could have been ticketed. It was just a joke and I fully intended to fight it. In fact, I videotaped 71 cars making the turn – 68 of which were "illegal". But, before I did the research, I paid the ticket and then planned to appeal using my video evidence.

Kansas law says that if you pay a fine, you are essentially admitting guilt and there can be no appeal. So, that became my new battle. I fought that by the argument that I should have been told before I paid the fine that I was abdicating my right to appeal. I likened it to being read your Miranda Rights – that you shouldn't be required to know what your rights were ahead of time. I lost that case in the District Court, so I appealed to the Kansas Court of Appeals – which is just below the Kansas Supreme Court. I represented myself because I thought I was smart enough to make the argument – and I still do. But, the Court of Appeals basically waved me off and sided with the city. I honestly think if I had an attorney, I could have affected the way that process was handled in the future. But, I had my fun.

I've only taken an illegal drug once in my life. It was 11PM on a Sunday night and I was going to drive back from western Kansas to my home in Topeka because I had to go to work the next day at 8AM. The problem was that it was a five-hour drive and I was very worried about falling asleep at the wheel. I don't even recall knowing about No Doze or any such thing in those days. This was in 1979.

But a person who will remain nameless gave me one or two (don't remember) "speed" pills. I'm probably not even using the right terminology. I believe they were amphetamines. They worked perfectly! I never noticed anything out of the ordinary, only that I was never even remotely tired at the wheel. I don't think it is over-exaggerating to say taking speed may have saved my life that night.

I can't imagine driving drunk or buying and using illegal drugs or committing robbery or anything else where the consequences could mean jail time. Having to look over one's shoulder seems like it would be a horrible way to live. Even though I was almost always poor before I got married in 1981, I never considered doing anything illegal. Whether that was due to my parents or not, I don't know.

When you spend your junior high and high school years living out in the country with little way to interact with kids in town after school or on weekends, it greatly reduces the chances of getting into trouble. So, although I hated those years in western Kansas growing up, it's probably true that my odds of ever doing anything serious against the law were also reduced. And, for that, I'm thankful.

My Thoughts

Martin has been a law abiding individual, and he has never taken illegal drugs (with that one tiny exception). One fact to note is that his father punished him for stealing money from his mother with a belt. It seems, then, that Martin's father used physical punishment, but that was not unusual in those days (and maybe even not today in some families).

Chapter 31

Extra Information

Although I have reproduced much of Martin's essays on his website, he has many other essays on the website, most of which have very little personal information. However, occasionally, he gives us some additional information. For example, he does mention occasional business ventures. In the early 1980s, he was involved with a satellite television company. His interested started with his friend Charles from high school days when they devised two devices to help those who sold and those who purchased satellite systems. One device located satellites, and the other device located sources of microwave interference. Both devices sold well. He, along with some partners, started a satellite television company in 1983 in Topeka, Kansas, that did well in the early 1980s until content providers began to use scramblers to prevent people getting the programs free. Martin left the company, but he notes that he tended to operate on three to four years cycles, changing jobs that often.

Martin was quite gifted in in his construction activities. He mentions that he worked in construction at one point in his life, and he gives examples of a scale model of the Hebrew Tabernacle (discussed in the Old Testament) that he built, a playground for his step-daughters that he built in their backyard (of which he was very proud), and the remodeling he did on the house he bought with his first wife, Chris.

He mentions having a real estate license and selling houses briefly in 1976 and being heavily involved in investing at another point., and then, in the late 1980s, produced three editions of a book on basketball called *Basketball Heaven,* a book for basketball fans similar to Bill James's books on baseball. He devised efficiency ratings for teams and players, and the book was very successful. But Martin lost interest in continually revising and updating the book for later editions, and he went back to the television company working in the security division.

In the year 2000, Martin joined the *Kansas City Star* to work on their statistics pages in the sports section. He then began a blog on the newspaper's website and, when he left the papers 18 months before his suicide, he re-created the blog as www.SportsInReview.com. Martin illustrates his obsessiveness when he notes that he wrote an entry for the newspaper blog for 653 consecutive days, sometimes two each day, only cutting back 18 months before his suicide when he realized that he had much to do to prepare for his suicide. In many activities in his life, Martin shows an obsessiveness, which he admits, but it is important to note that his obsessiveness was focused on productive activities. He did not clean his house obsessively to the detriment of his career or relationships, or wash his hands fifty times a day, as those with obsessive-compulsive disorder might do. His obsessions bore fruit. For example, people in the know (at ESPN, for example) rated *Basketball Heaven* as a superb book.

He mentions many activities that he was engaged in, particularly during his second marriage with Teri, including poker, singing in the choir, playing chess, (especially against the early computer chess programs), bicycling (with his wife and with neighbors), paintball, canoeing, bowling, and barbeque contests.

Martin also mentions some fears. He decided to never leave America for vacations because Americans become targets and get kidnapped and arrested abroad. He mentions stepping across into Canada for a few seconds in the way that I have stepped across the DMZ in Korea into North Korea for a few seconds, although North Korea is very different from Canada!!!!!! He disliked flying, although he did take airplane flights when necessary. In 1998, he purchased gold and silver coins in case there was an economic collapse in the United States.

Finally, despite the way he seems to portray himself as an independent person, and indeed asserts frequently that he is, he talks of friends, wives, step-children and neighbors. He mentions moving to Florida in 2004 and missing everyone back home in Kansas. He talks of socializing with his sister and brother, including a time when his brother bought tickets to a World Series baseball game for the two of them.

Part 3: Conclusion

Chapter 32

Jo Roman

Before discussing the rationality of Martin's decision to die by suicide, I would like to present another example of an individual who seems to have made a rational decision to die by suicide, but for a more conventional reason. Jo Roman decided to hasten her death by suicide in the face of advanced cancer. She wrote a book about her life and about this decision, and it seems to me to be a good example of a rational suicide.

Jo Roman spent part of her life considering whether rational suicide existed and, after she decided that it was, thinking of how society might assist those who wished to commit suicide to do so in a dignified manner. When she was sixty-one, in March 1978, Jo was diagnosed with advanced breast cancer, and so she killed herself in line with the principles that she had earlier worked out.

Early Life

Jo was born on February 3, 1917, at her parents' home in Cambridge, Massachusetts. She was named in honor of the doctor who delivered her -- Mary. Her parents had already lost a girl in infancy. Jo had a brother four years older (Fred) and, later, a younger brother.

When Jo was born, Jo's father, Charles Clodfelter, called Claude by her mother, was 42 and a minister in the Swedenborgian Church. Her mother, Adeline, was 27. Claude was born on a farm in Missouri but had left to become a minister. A few months after Jo's birth, the family moved to Fall River, Massachusetts, to start a mission there among the Catholics. Although her parents treated Fred normally, they were extremely overprotective of Jo. They did not let her play with or talk to other children except when supervised by her parents and, until the age eleven, Jo was never out of the sight of her parents, brother, or parent-approved adult. Her mother's discipline was harsh and her rules rigid. There were daily spankings, and Jo's mouth was washed out with soap if she said the wrong thing. Her father did sometimes take Jo with him on visits to parishioners, but by the age of ten Jo had decided that God was a figment of man's imagination.

The family moved to a new parish in 1928, in Lancaster, Pennsylvania. By now, Jo knew how to handle her parents by appearing to be the obedient girl they desired. They permitted her to play with other children at her home (but not at their homes), and Jo developed a double life, slipping secretly into the homes of her friends and developing her own self. She decided that she did not like the name Mary and chose Mary Jo Anne. She registered at school as Mary Joanne, and graduated as Mary Joan, which confused her parents. She persuaded them to call her Mary Jo, and later to drop the Mary.

Jo went to college at Millersville State Teacher's College where she developed a good friend, Mary Butts, and fell in love with a boy who hadn't finished high school and who worked in a wholesale hardware firm. Jo's parents wanted them to postpone a marriage, so Jo and Bill married secretly in March 1937 and continued to live apart. Jo graduated and worked as a grade school teacher, while Bill graduated from the Wharton School at the University of Pennsylvania in 1939. They now had an official wedding ceremony and moved in together. A son Tom was born in 1940 and a daughter Timmy in 1942.

In March 1943, on the sixth anniversary of their marriage, Bill had to have a hernia operation, and he died of a heart attack during the surgery. After a period of grieving, Jo took the children off to Alaska where she worked as an interior designer. She quickly met the Governor's wife there, who introduced Jo into social life of the Governor. Jo's life blossomed, and she fell in love with the Governor's aide, Warren Caro. However, Jo was often exhausted, plagued by insomnia, and found herself wishing to be dead whenever she wasn't preoccupied with her work. She felt that she was a poor mother to her children, and she decided to send the children to live with her college friend, Mary, who was now married to a minister and who was unable to have children. Eventually, Mary adopted the children, but Jo appears to have kept in contact with her children and to have established good relationships with them.

Jo left Alaska early in 1946 and visited her parents and her children in Pennsylvania. She moved on to New York City to develop her relationship with Warren and, after meeting Robert Laidlaw, a psychiatrist interested in marriage counseling, got involved in the newly-formed American Association of Marriage Counselors. There she met Ernest Groves who arranged for Jo to be admitted to Duke University as a graduate student in the department he was starting there. Groves died in August, before the semester had started, and Jo spent a year in the psychology department, which had a curriculum she hated but which, with the aide of two fellow students, Sam and Bob, she survived for one year. She was quite ill during the year, with heavy menstrual flows, a hysterectomy, and an infection of the ears and sinuses. Jo became Bob's lover, despite remaining involved with Warren who was in New York, but by the end of the year decided that she wanted to end her existence. She overdosed on Seconal, but survived. Jo said that she never again felt suicidal.

Despite passing her exams, she quit the psychology department at Duke University and moved back to New York. She worked for a while at the Margaret Sanger Research Bureau, which was conducting pioneering work on birth control and family planning, and she married Warren in November 1947,

Jo went into an orthodox psychoanalysis and, although her analyst died after two and a half years, she continued her analysis with another analyst, completing five years. She earned a master's degree in psychiatric social work. However, after five years of marriage, she decided that she and Warren were not compatible, and so they divorced.

Two years later, in 1952, in the course of her work, she met Mel Roman, a psychologist. Mel was married with a three year old, but unhappy. After Mel separated and divorced his wife, he and Jo got involved. Jo was concerned that Mel was ten years younger than she was and that she had been alone for only two years, but they married and remained happy together.

Jo worked for Hillside Hospital, the psychiatric clinic of New York City's Domestic Relations Court (where she had met Mel), and then the University Settlement House. After Mel had a heart attack, he cut back his hours of work, and they established an apartment with an office nearby and started a private practice. They ventured into art, starting with "interaction paintings" (on which both of them worked). They vacationed on Cape Cod, renting a house for the summers. In 1963, they went down to Mississippi to work for the Medical Committee of Human Rights.

They eventually renovated a row of brownstones on the West Side which they turned into a co-op and in which they had an apartment and studio. Jo developed the idea of "touch boxes," whose interiors could not be seen but which had to be explored by hand. Mel got involved with Paolo Soleri and the plans for building ecologically sound communities in Arizona.

A neighbor in the brownstones, Jochen Seidel, an artist, decided that he had completed his life as an artist and had no wish to live any more. He made several suicide attempts, and Jo "saved" him on two occasions. Finally, in 1971, he hanged himself successfully, and this made Jo think more about rational suicide.

In 1975, at the age of fifty-eight, Jo began to think about how long she would live and how she might like to die. She considered that a life span of 75 years was sufficient, for after that she might well become ill, feeble and decrepit.[1] She planned to commit suicide in 1992, starting a folder about the "project" and adding notes to the folder irregularly. She began to raise the topic of rational suicide with friends and to plan how society might accommodate those who wished to commit suicide. She called her project *Exit House*.

When she discussed her ideas with Mel, he was disturbed. He was distressed by the thought of losing Jo when she was 75 and he was only 65, and the discussions created a good deal of conflict. Mel's mother died of cancer in early 1976. He saw how the doctors and family conspired to keep the information from her that she had cancer, and he saw how she suffered as the cancer killed her. Finally, Mel asked the doctor to let his mother die, but it still seemed to him that Jo was abandoning him.

In 1997, Jo and Mel decided to spend two months of the summer of 1978 apart, to pursue their own projects. However, in late 1977, Jo's daughter Timmy developed breast cancer. Jo helped her through the treatment, and then in March 1978 Jo was diagnosed with advanced breast cancer, and she advanced the planned date for her suicide.

Jo kept the information from Mel and others, and she even tried chemotherapy without telling anyone. But eventually the nausea became too severe, and she told Mel in June, 1978. Finally, Jo decided on one year of life of good quality without chemotherapy rather than two years of hell with chemotherapy. In retrospect, Jo considered the ten months she spent trying chemotherapy and suffering the resulting debilitation to have been a waste of time.

Jo killed herself on June 10, 1979, with an overdose of Seconal.

[1] Fifteen years longer than Martin felt was enough.

Guidelines for Rational Suicide

In the preparations for her suicide, Jo, with the assistance of her husband, Mel, reached out to her family and friends. She discussed it in depth with everyone, she wrote her obituary, and she began to write her book, *Exit House*, which would be her legacy to others and which was published after her death. As the final section of this book, Jo brought together her interest in rational suicide, her experiences as a social worker and her interior design skills to design an Exit House for the future, complete with a description of the legal basis, services provided, and even floor plans for the suites which the suicides would occupy. Alfred Nobel (after whom the Nobel Prizes are named), who had proposed such an idea a hundred years earlier, would have been very pleased!

Jo brought up the topic of her suicide with doctors and eventually found one who advised her so that she could decide on a lethal dose of Seconal accompanied by a champagne toast. One doctor offered to give her a lethal injection, and two nurses offered to help with the suicide, but Jo declined their assistance. Other doctors offered to sign her death certificate with a cause other than suicide, offers she also declined. She accumulated the Seconal as a sleeping pill over several years, and friends added to her supply. However, Jo felt strongly that a safe and effective "exit pill" should be devised and made available in drug stores for those who wish to kill themselves. The availability of such a pill might prevent many impulsive suicides since these individuals would know that the option for suicide was readily available, and it might also prevent "violent" and bloody suicides.

Jo wished that rational suicides had the opportunity to have a medical assistant to help with the death itself, a practical assistant to help suicidal individuals think through and manage the practical issues of ending a life (such as wills and insurance), a protective assistant to prevent people stumbling across you as you lay dying and "saving" you, and personal assistants to be with you on your journey. The last of these is possible. Jo developed her own circle and urged rational suicides to start this early on in the process. Discuss your plans with friends and family and see which of those would assist you. Jo's circle grew to one hundred, and she left a letter for three hundred people. Jo's hope was that such circles could arise which were not centered around only one individual, but whose goal could be to be there for anyone in the circle.

In the week before her suicide, Jo and Mel talked -- "marathon sessions" is how Mel described them -- and they met with family members and close friends. The times were full of tears and laughter. For the final weekend, they made a film in which Jo, Mel and their intimate friends discussed the issues and Jo's impending suicide. Jo also wrote a letter which was mailed to some three hundred friends and family members on the day that she killed herself. Mel notes that the loss of his wife was painful, but the discussions and anticipatory grieving helped him recover from the loss. He felt enriched by the experience, as did many of Jo's friends.

Jo Roman's suicide fits the accepted form of rational suicide. She has terminal cancer. She has tried treatment and rejected it because it will seriously impair her remaining months of life. She has thought through her decision for many years, both intellectually at first, and then as a personal dilemma. She is not depressed and seems to be at peace with her decision. She has discussed it with her husband and significant others, and they appear to have agreed with her that her decision is the correct one, or at least one they find reasonable and acceptable.

Chapter 33

Was Martin's Decision to Die by Suicide Rational?

This is the question for us to consider, the reason for this book. But let me address another issue first. Was his death an appropriate death?

Was Martin's Death Appropriate?

In Chapter 3, I discussed various criteria for a death to be appropriate, but we should remember that there may be other criteria. However, Martin's death by suicide is appropriate on many of the criteria that I listed in Chapter 3. First, in line with Weisman and Hackett, he faced death with no anxiety. It served to reduce the conflicts and problems in his life (in his case, over aging), and there no relationships that he needed to continue.

In his eyes, the timing of his death was ideal. He died "at the top" rather than hanging on too long, and he avoided the pitfalls and perils of a decline in old age. He played a role in his own death, a critical factor for those for whom autonomy in choices is important. His biological, psychological and social death occurred at the same time. True, shooting himself damaged his bodily integrity, but most of us will die without bodily integrity. I've had three major surgeries, and I have a pacemaker. My bodily integrity was lost many years ago!

Therefore, I would judge Martin's death to be, not only appropriate, but more appropriate than the majority of deaths.

Was Martin's Choice Rational?

Despite my criticisms of psychiatry and psychiatrists in Chapter 4, I have to discuss whether Martin had a diagnosable psychiatric disorder and, if so, was it severe enough to impair his judgment.

Any psychiatrist reading about Martin will know that he died by suicide. This knowledge will bias their judgment. Ideally, they should read his life story with the indication (and hints) that he died by suicide removed. Only then should they diagnose him. I mentioned in Chapter 4 that Eli Robins and his colleagues judged every suicide in their sample to have a psychiatric disorder, but they had knowledge of the cause of death. That knowledge renders their study invalid.

What symptoms do we find in Martin? Remember that I have not edited the essays above except to correct no more than half a dozen misspellings. He writes well, coherently, argues his point intelligently, and is witty. Intellectually, he seems to be, not just fine, but outstanding. Schizophrenia is defined by the symptoms of hallucinations, delusions, inappropriate emotions, strange postures and gesture, language that is difficult to follow (commonly called *schizophrenese*), and disorientation. Martin shows none of these psychotic symptoms. What about the affective disorders, that is, severe depression (major depressive disorder) and manic-depression (bipolar disorder)? He says that he does not consider himself to be depressed, but merely sad. I noted earlier (in Chapter 4) that Eric Wilson has argued that we should accept the melancholy that is going to be present in everyone's life.

My conclusion is that Martin did not have the most severe psychiatric disorders – the psychoses.

In the old days, there used to be an umbrella term for the moderate psychiatric disorders – the neuroses. It is still a useful term and includes anxiety disorders (phobias, obsessive-compulsive disorders, panic attacks, etc.), dissociative disorders (amnesia and multiple personality), and conversion disorders (paralyses and sensory losses such as blindness and deafness, with no physiological cause). Although Martin described himself as obsessive, his obsessiveness does not impair his life. A truly obsessive individual may, for example, wash his hands hundreds of times a day in case he has bacteria on them. He may be unable to work and have meaningful relationships with others. Martin's obsessiveness (mainly about his work and eating habits) is common. After all, this book by me is being written by someone who has over 2,500 scholarly publications. Obsessiveness can be productive if it is work-oriented rather than hygiene-oriented! It should be remembered that, although we often call our weird friends *neurotic*, true neuroses severely impair your life. Martin's life has not been impaired much at all. And lest you bring up his two marriages, I have been happily married for over 25 years – after two "failed" marriages.

Therefore, Martin does not seem to have a moderate or severe psychiatric disorder.

This brings us to the mildest psychiatric disorders, the personality disorders. Personality disorders are chronic maladaptive life styles. This is what almost all of us have if we do not have a psychosis or neurosis. All of us could have had a much more successful life if only we didn't……Fill in the blank. We could have a more successful career, a more fulfilling marriage, a greater feeling of well-being, etc. Thus, a personality disorder does not mean that you are incompetent and unable to make rational decisions.

Martin tells us that he is somewhat obsessive, and I have commented that he seems to be narcissistic. However, in my opinion, these tendencies, which in the extreme, can be considered to be personality disorders, are mild in Martin, and they do not seem to impair his decision-making.

I, therefore, judge that Martin is not impaired by psychiatric symptoms or disorders.

What about the other criteria for irrationality that I listed in Chapter 2. Yes, his decision is statistically rare. Is it motivated by unconscious desires? Probably, but as I noted in Chapter 2, if you follow Freudian theory, every decision we make is motivated in part by unconscious desires. Is Martin maximizing utility (in economic terms) or his satisfaction (in psychological terms)? In his eyes, he is.

What our decision about Martin's rationality comes down to is whether we think his premises, his assumptions, are rational.

Unlike Jo Roman (in Chapter 31 above), Martin does not a medical illness, let alone a terminal medical illness. Therefore, Martin does not have the "acceptable" reason for suicide, that of avoiding more physical pain, in which the choice of suicide merely shortens one's life by a few months. Martin put witty quotes throughout his essays, so perhaps I may be permitted one here, which I heard from R. D. Laing (an existential psychiatrist).

Life is a Sexually Transmitted Disease with 100% Mortality

Death is inevitable. We all will die. Martin has shortened his life, but by how much we do not know.

David Burns (1980) described ten types of irrational thinking:

- *In all-or-nothing thinking,* the person sees things in black and white categories. If your performance is not perfect, you are a failure.
- In *overgeneralization,* the client makes unjustified generalizations on the basis of one incident. For example, a single failure leads the client to believe that he will never succeed at anything.
- *Mental filter* involves picking out negative details and dwelling on them exclusively.
- *Disqualifying the positive* involves rejecting positive experiences because, for some reason, they don't count.
- When clients *jump to conclusions,* they incorrectly read the mind of others (without checking with those others whether their conclusion is correct or not), and they predict the future incorrectly (usually pessimistically).
- In *magnification* (or *catastrophizing),* the client exaggerates the significance of an event. If you fear dying, you may interpret every unpleasant sensation as a fatal disease.
- In *emotional reasoning,* clients assume that, because they feel it is, it must be true.
- *Should statements,* such as "I must," "I ought," and "I should" lead to guilt. They should be replaced with "It would be nice if I..."
- *Labeling* is an extreme form of overgeneralization. Others are rarely as evil as you think they are, and you are not as bad as you think you are. For example, calling others "bastards" or yourself a "loser" leads to strong negative emotions.
- In *personalization* you see yourself as the cause of some negative outcome when, in reality, you were not the only, or even the primary, cause.

Martin shows some of these traits. His fears of growing old and the extreme mental decline that he anticipates fit into the categories of catastrophizing, jumping to conclusions, mental filter and all-or-nothing thinking. Obviously, I did not know Martin personally, and so I cannot know how bad his mental decline was. I have referred to his memory lapses as "senior moments." As far as I can tell from his essay, they seemed minor, and the newspaper headlines that I read announcing that Martin killed himself because of dementia seem to be gross exaggerations. But I wasn't there. However, I can be sure, because I read his essays, that, right up to his last days, he was writing well-constructed, well-argued, coherent and witty essays. This was not someone with dementia.

Unlike legislators in Oregon and other states that have legalized assisted-suicide in cases of terminal illness, I do not see physical pain and suffering as "real," whereas mental pain is "not real." Mental pain, what Edwin Shneidman (1996) has called *psychache*, can be as bad, if not worse, than physical pain. However, Martin does not seem to be depressed or anxious. He does not seem to have psychache right now. He meets one of the criteria for rationality of not being swayed by emotions, but only by thoughts.

Perhaps our judgment of the rationality of his premises (or assumptions) comes down to our subjective opinion. For what reasons would we choose to die by suicide? Would I choose suicide if I had a terminal illness? Perhaps. Would you? Would I immolate myself as a political protest against the government? Never! Would we choose suicide to avoid experiencing mental and physical decline in the next ten or twenty years? I would not, but then I have lots of projects and goals, like writing this book and taking another cruise with my wife. Martin has few goals left, if any.

Therefore, although I would not choose suicide for the same reasons as Martin (and indeed, at age 71, I have not), I cannot find any evidence to label his decision as irrational.

Chapter 34

Final Thoughts

In this final chapter, I would like to do two things. First, James Werth, a psychologist who supports the legalization of assisted suicide in the United States, has proposed criteria for rational suicide. I will review his criteria and criticize them as too restrictive. Second, I will propose how, in this modern age, clinicians should counseling those individuals who are contemplating suicide.

Werth (1998) proposed the following criteria for rational suicide:

1. The person considering suicide has an unremitting "hopeless" condition. "Hopeless" conditions include, but are not necessarily limited to, terminal illness, severe physical and/or psychological pain, physically or mentally debilitating and/or deteriorating conditions, or quality of life no longer acceptable to the individual.
2. The person makes the decision as a free choice (i.e., is not pressured by others to choose suicide).
3. The person has engaged in a sound decision- making process. This process includes the following:

    *   Consultation with a mental health professional who can make an assessment of mental competence (which would include the absence of treatable major depression);
    *   Non-impulsive consideration of all alternatives;
    *   Consideration of the congruence of the act with one's personal values;
    *   Consultation with objective others (e.g., medical and religious professionals) and with significant others.

These are not bad, but I would object to three of the requirements. James Werth is a psychologist who is concerned with gaining public and government approval of a less restrictive attitude toward assisted-suicide, and so he is proposing criteria that might gain acceptance in these circles, as it has in Oregon. In this book, I do not have to be as politically careful.

First, criterion number 1 is too restrictive as a general criterion for rational suicide. To be sure, for official assisted suicide policies, only such a restrictive criterion as this would win government approval today.

But I do not think that terminal illnesses and extreme pain are the only conditions under which a suicide may be considered to be rational. An unacceptable quality of life is a good criterion, but I doubt that even Werth would judge Martin's quality of life to be unacceptable given his previous list of conditions (terminal illness and extreme pain). I would allow individuals to decide about the quality of their lives even though, to others, the quality might appear to be fine.

Pridmore (2009) set out to find individuals who chose suicide because of the predicament they found themselves and who were not psychiatrically disturbed. Aside from Ajax, a Greek mythical individual, and Brutus who conspired to kill Julius Caesar in ancient Rome, Pridmore mentioned the mayor of Leipzig, Alfred Freyburg, a Nazi, who died by suicide after the city surrendered to American troops, and General Walter Donnicke who died by suicide in Leipzig that same day.

He also thought that Thich Quang Duc, a Buddhist monk who immolated himself in 1963 in Saigon (Vietnam) to protest the government oppression of Buddhists, and Bud Dwyer, a former treasurer of the state of Pennsylvania, who had just been convicted and faced a prison sentence, met this criterion. Whether these particular individuals meet Pridmore's criteria (that is, free from mental illness, but in a serious predicament), may be disputed, but Pridmore's suggestion of this type of suicide is intriguing.

I also object to criterion 3a, as you might expect. "Mental health professionals" is a vague term, but it includes psychiatrists and those who follow the psychiatric model (as do many social workers and psychologists). As you saw in Chapter 4, I am strongly critical of this model.

Such consultants would be biased and unfit to make an assessment of mental competence. If this criterion is absolutely necessary, then a group of unbiased mental health professionals who are neither biased toward encouraging suicide, nor biased against preventing every suicide, must be identified for such assessments. I doubt that many could be found among the psychiatric profession.

Similarly, in 3e, I would remove "medical and religious professionals" unless one can identify those without bias for or against suicide. When I mentioned to a colleague once the problem of finding unbiased counselors with whom to discuss suicide, she suggested that those engaged in hospice care might be the best. Since they deal with people who are dying and often contemplating suicide, they are made less anxious and are less threatened by discussing this choice with others.

The other criteria seem fine.

Why is there such opposition to suicide, even rational suicide? Sigmund Freud noted that we impose moral taboos only on those behaviors that we are tempted (consciously or unconsciously) to do ourselves.

The opposition to suicide then suggests that we are continually fighting our own suicidal impulses. Perhaps all of those who study suicide as scholars are defending against our suicidal impulses (conscious and unconscious) using the defense mechanism of intellectualization (which gives us an illusory sense of control), and those who devote their efforts to preventing suicide are similarly defending against their own suicidal impulses. How might we counseling a suicidal individual if we want to be free from bias? The following is from an essay I wrote a few years ago on this issue (Lester, 1995).

Counseling the Suicidal Individual in the Modern Age

How then should a counselor approach a person who is seriously considering suicide? An obvious first step is to do what any good counselor does, that is, to act as a person-centered counselor – actively listen to the client (Gordon, 1970). The client's situation needs to be explored and the client's thoughts and feelings about the situation expressed. If family therapy is possible, then the position of significant others in the family must be explored until at some point the situation is clear both to the client and to the counselor.

The second step is for the counselor to explore the suicidogenic factors. What stresses has the client experienced (physical illnesses, losses, etcetera)? What psychological factors are present, such as psychiatric disorder, depression, cognitive distortions, and so on? What is the social situation of the client, and what are reasonable expectations for the future? Part of the task here is to educate the client about suicide – what we know of the causes and concomitant characteristics of the suicidal crisis.

The third step is to discuss options. The presence of a severe illness does not argue for or against suicide. If the client has not tried treatment yet, then trying treatment is a possible first option. Then the counselor and client can continue to meet to discuss the effects of the treatment. For example, Abbie Hoffman, a probable manic-depressive, did not like the effects of lithium on his body. He tried to medicate himself with Prozac and Valium. His eventual suicide may suggest that his preferred medications were not appropriate, but discussion of all of the decisions that he made with a counselor may have enabled his choices to be better informed choices.

Each time that the client makes a decision, then the counselor's task is to help the client carry out that decision. If the decision is to try a new treatment, then the counselor will help the client go through the process. If the decision is to refuse treatment, and even to terminate life, then the counselor will help the client to carry out these decisions. The client should be reminded that decisions made are only decisions at that point in time and that decisions can be changed. A decision to undergo treatment can be reversed; a decision to die by suicide can, up to the final moments, be reversed.

The best framework for a counselor with these goals is *Direct-Decision Therapy*, proposed by Harold Greenwald (1973). Direct-decision therapy focuses on the decisions that clients make. The task of the therapist is to help clients make decision and to help clients carry out these decisions. Clients choose their problems, according to Greenwald. They choose to be afraid of heights, to be depressed, or to have an unhappy marriage. Once the therapist has helped the client become aware of these decisions, the next task is to identify the circumstances in which the decision was made. After this is done, the decision no longer appears to be irrational.

For example, a child may have grown up with a depressed parent. The child may have noticed that when he or she is sick, the parent becomes less lethargic and takes care of the child. The child may then experiment and discover that, when he or she is upset, the parent also behaves less depressed in order to care for the child's feelings. Thus, the child may decide to cope with a depressed parent by being more depressed than the parent. While this may be a bad strategy for an adult interacting with other adults, it is not a bad solution for a young child trying to cope with a depressed parent, for young children have fewer strategies available to them.

Greenwald next helps the client to assess the advantages and the disadvantages of the decisions they have made in the past, and this must be done without criticizing the client. Then the client must devise or be presented with alternative decisions, and for each of these the client must be helped to assess the positive and negative gain. Clients must be helped to become aware of alternatives and their consequences.

However, it is the client, and the client alone, who must decide which alternative to choose, Once the client has chosen, then the therapist's final task is to help the client make that decision and accomplish his or her goals, although the therapist should make sure that the client realizes that a decision has to be reaffirmed continually and that decisions can be changed.

In the examples given by Greenwald, it is clear that the therapist does not evaluate the decisions as appropriate or inappropriate, with the proviso that some actions may be illegal, such as murder and other felonies. It is the client's life, and the client must make and live with the decision, not the therapist. Once the client has made a decision and realizes the consequences (both positive and negative), it is the therapist's responsibility to help the client achieve his or her goals.

Let me emphasize this point. Direct Decision Therapy does not impose values on the client. The client is free to choose whatever he or she wants, and Greenwald's goal is awareness in terms of the choices made, the context in which these choices were made, and the payoff's. Only in this way can people be assisted in making rational decisions about suicide.

References

Aarons, D. (1985). *The Inman diary*. Cambridge, MA: Harvard University Press.

Angell, M. (2012a). The epidemic of mental illness: Why? www.nybooks.com/articles/archives/2011/jun/23/epidemic-mental-illness-why/?pagination=false

Angell, M. (2012b). The illusions of psychiatry. www.nybooks.com/articles/archives/2011/jul/14/illusions-of-psychiatry/?pagination=false

American Psychiatric Association. (2013). *Diagnostic and statistical manual of mental disorders, fifth edition, DSM-5*. Washington, DC: American Psychiatric Publishing.

Anon. (August 3, 2013). Locked in. *The Economist, 408(8847),* 24-25.

Baum, R. (1974). *Logic*. New York: Holt, Rinehart & Winston.

Beauchamp, T., & Childress, J. (1979). *Principles of biomedical ethics*. New York: Oxford University Press.

Beck, A. T., Ward, C H., Mendelson, M., Mock, J. E., & Erbaugh, J. K. (1962). Reliability of psychiatric diagnoses. *American Journal of Psychiatry, 119,* 351-357.

Binswanger, L. (1958). The case of Ellen West. In R. May, E. Angel & H. F. Ellenberger (Eds.) *Existence*, pp. 237-364. New York: Basic Books.

Blachly, P. H. (1971). Can organ transplantation provide an altruistic-expiatory alternative to suicide? *Life-Threatening Behavior, 1,* 5-9.

Burns, D. D. (1980). *Feeling good*. New York: Morrow.

Cairns, R., Maddock, C., Buchanan, A., David, A., Hayward, P., Richardson, G., Szmukler, G., & Hotopf, M. (2005). Prevalence and predictors of mental incapacity in psychiatric in-patients. *British Journal of Psychiatry, 187,* 379-385.

Carlat, D. (2010). *Unhinged*. New York: Free Press.

Chelminski, I., Ferrarto, F. R., Petros, T. V., & Plaud, J. j. (1999). An analysis of the "eveningness-morningness" dimension in "depressive" college students. *Journal of Affective Disorders, 52,* 19-29.

Clarke, R.V., & Lester, D. (1989). *Suicide: Closing the exits*. New York: Spring-Verlag.

Diekstra, R. F. W. (1995). Dying in dignity. *Psychiatry & Clinical Neurosciences,* 49(Supplement 1), S139-S148.

Ellis, A. (1973). *Humanistic psychotherapy*. New York: Julian.

Engel, S. M. (1986). *With good reason*. New York: St. Martins.

Gay, P. (1988). *Freud*. New York: Norton.

Goldstein, K. (1940). *Human nature in the light of psychopathology*. Cambridge, MA: Harvard University Press.

Gordon, T. (1970). *Parent effectiveness training*. New York: Wyden.

Greenwald, H. (1973). *Direct-decision therapy*. San Diego, CA: Edits.

Hauerwas, S. (1981). Rational suicide and reasons for living. *Progress in Clinical & Biological Research*, 50, 185-199.

Hewitt, J. (2010). Schizophrenia, mental capacity, and rational suicide. *Theoretical Medicine & Bioethics, 31*, 63-77.

Hewitt, J. (2013). Why are people with mental illness excluded from the rational suicide debate? *International Journal of Law & Psychiatry, 36,* 358-365.

Hutchings, D., Simpson, R., Stauffer, R., & Wahl, D. (2007). Aesthetics, death, and landmark structures. *Journal of Architectural Engineering, 13,* 1-8.

Jackson, J. E. (1992). "After a while no one believes you:" Real and unreal pain. In M. J. D. Good, P. E. Brodwin, B. J. Good & A. Kleinman (Eds.), *Pain as human experience*, pp. 138-168. Berkeley, CA: University of California Press.

Joiner, T. E. (2005). *Why people die by suicide*. Cambridge, MA: Harvard University Press.

Kalish, R. A. (1985). *Death, grief, and caring relationships*. Monterey, CA: Brooks/Cole.

Kemp, R., Chua, S., McKenna, P., & David, A. (1997). Reasoning and delusions. *British Journal of Psychiatry, 170,* 398-405.

Kim, C. H., Jayathilake, K., & Meltzer, H. Y. (2003). Hopelessness, neurocognitive function, and insight in schizophrenia. *Schizophrenia Research, 60,* 71-80.

Kirsch, I. (2010). *The Emperor's new drugs*. New York: Basic Books.

Leeman, C. P. (2009). Distinguishing among irrational suicide and other forms of hastened death. *Psychosomatics, 50,* 185-191.

Leenaars, A. A. (1986). A brief note on latent content in suicide notes. *Psychological Reports*, 59, 640-642.

Leenaars, A. A., & Lester, D. (Eds.) (1996). *Suicide and the unconscious*. Northvale, NJ: Jason Aronson.

Lester, D. (1991). The study of suicidal lives. *Suicide & Life-Threatening Behavior*, 21, 164-173.

Lester, D. (1995). Counseling the suicidal person in the modern age. *Crisis Intervention, 2,* 159-163.

Lester, D. (1996-1997). AIDS and rational suicide. *Omega*, 34, 333-336.

Lester, D. (2003). *Fixin' to die*. Amityville, NY: Baywood.

Lester, D. (2005). *Suicide and the Holocaust*. Hauppauge, NY: Nova Science.

Lester, D. (2006). Sex differences in completed suicide by schizophrenic patients. *Suicide & Life-Threatening Behavior, 36,* 50-56.

Lester, D. (2010). The reasons for suicide. *Death Studies, 34,* 54-70.

Linehan, M. M., Goodstein, J. L., Nielsen, S. L., & Chiles, J. A. (1983). Reasons for staying alive when you are thinking of killing yourself. *Journal of Consulting & Clinical Psychology, 51,* 276-286.

Margolis, J. (1975). *Negativities*. Columbus, OH: Merrill.

Menninger, K. (1938). *Man against himself*. New York: Harcourt, Brace & World.

Owen, G., Cutting, J., & David, A. (2007). Are people with schizophrenia more logical than health volunteers? *British Journal of Psychiatry, 191,* 453-454.

Owen, G., Richardson, G., David, A., Szmukler, G., Hayward, P., & Hotopf, M. (2008). Mental capacity to make decisions on treatment in people admitted to psychiatric hospitals. *British Medical journal, 337,* 40-42

Pompili, M., et al. (2007). Suicide risk in schizophrenia. *Annals of General Psychiatry, 6,* #10.

Pretzel, P. W. (1968). Philosophical and ethical considerations of suicide prevention. *Bulletin of Suicidology*, July, 30-38.

Pridmore, S. (2009). Predicament suicide. *Australasian Psychiatry, 17,* 112-116.

Rankin, A. (2011). *Seppuku.* New York: Kodansha International.

Robins, E. (1981). *The final months.* New York: Oxford University Press.

Roman, J. (1980). *Exit house.* New York: Seaview Books.

Sandifer, M., Horden, A., Timbury, G., & Green, L. (1968). Psychiatric diagnosis. *British Journal of Psychiatry, 114,* 1-9.

Shneidman, E. S. (1967). Sleep and self-destruction. In E. S. Shneidman (Ed.) *Essays in self-destruction*, pp. 510-539. New York: Science House.

Shneidman, E. S. (1970). Content analysis of suicidal logic. In E. S. Shneidman, N. L. Farberow, & R. E. Litman (Eds.) *The psychology of suicide*, pp. 73-93. New York: Science House.

Shneidman, E. S. (1982a). On "Therefore I must kill myself." *Suicide & Life Threatening Behavio*r, 12, 52-55.

Shneidman, E. S. (1982b). The suicidal logic of Cesare Pavese. *Journal of the American Academy of Psychoanalysis*, 10, 547-563.

Shneidman, E. S. (1996). *The suicidal mind.* New York: Oxford University Press.

Shneidman, E. S., & Farberow, N. L. (1970). The logic of suicide. In E. S. Shneidman, N. L. Farberow, & R. E. Litman (Eds.) *The psychology of suicide*, pp. 63-71. New York: Science House.

Sullivan, M. (2001). Finding pain between mind and bodies. *Clinical Journal of Pain ,17,* 146-156.

Szasz, T. (1974). *The myth of mental illness.* New York: Harper & Row.

Temoche, A., Pugh, T. F., & MacMahon, B. (1964). Suicide rates among current and former mental institution patients. *Journal of Nervous & Mental Disease*, 138, 124-130.

Toman, W. (1960). *An introduction to the psychoanalytic theory of motivation.* New York: Pergamon.

Viscusi, W. k., (1984). *Cigarette taxation and the social consequences of smoking.* Cambridge, MA: National bureau of Economic Research.

Weisman, A., & Hackett, T. P. (1961). Predilection to death. *Psychosomatic Medicine, 23,* 232-256.

Werth, J. L. (1998). Using rational suicide as an intervention to prevent irrational suicide. *Crisis, 19,* 185-192.

Werth, J. L. (1996). *Rational suicide?* Washington, DC: Taylor & Francis.

Whitaker, R. (2010). *Anatomy of an epidemic.* New York: Crown.

Wilber, C. G. (1987). Some thoughts on suicide: is it logical? *American Journal of Forensic Medicine & Pathology*, 8, 302-308.

Wilson, E. G. (2008). *Against happiness: In praise of melancholy.* New York: Farrar, Straus & Giroux.

Wilson, S. T., & Amador, X. F. (2007). Awareness of illness and the risk of suicide in schizophrenia. In R. Tatarelli, M. Pompili & P. Girardi (Eds.), *Suicide in schizophrenia,* pp. 133-145. Hauppauge, NY: Nova Science.

Yang, B., & Lester, D. (2006). A prolegomenon to behavioral economic studies of suicide. In M. Altman (Ed.) *Handbook of contemporary behavioral economics*, pp. 543-559. Armonk, NY: M. E. Sharpe.

Yang, B., & Lester, D. (2007). Recalculating the economic cost of suicide. *Death Studies, 31,* 351-361.

Yeh, B. Y., & Lester, D. (1987). An economic model for suicide. In D. Lester, *Suicide as a learned behavior*, pp. 51-57. Springfield, IL: Charles Thomas.

Index

Hobart Mowrer, 47
hobby, 68
homes, 147
hopelessness, 3, 23, 24, 27, 46
hormones, 104
hospice, 8, 158
hospitalization, 26
house, 149, 150, 163
human, 5, 34, 61, 63, 78, 84, 129, 162
human behavior, 5
human experience, 162
humanistic psychology, 47
Hunter, 140
husband, 9, 10, 35, 150
hygiene, 154
hyperactivity, 113
hypersomnia, 22
hysterectomy, 148

I

ideal, 56, 57, 63, 77, 108, 117, 118, 123, 139, 153
identity, 98
Idio-logic, 11
illusions, 161
image, 38, 42, 91
imagination, 78, 147
imbalances, 22
IMO, 84, 120, 128, 129, 130
impulses, 158
impulsive, 7, 52, 120, 150, 157
income, 130
individuals, 4, 7, 8, 10, 12, 13, 19, 21, 24, 25, 26, 42, 47, 52, 57, 70, 120, 121, 150, 157, 158
industry, 23, 129, 130
infancy, 147
infection, 148
inheritance, 8
inmates, 6
innocence, 3
insane, 39, 134
insanity, 84, 140
insomnia, 22, 148
instinct, 41
integrity, 17, 153
intelligence, 24, 135
interference, 143
interpersonal relations, 6, 47, 121
interpersonal relationships, 6, 47, 121
intervention, 163
intrusions, ix, 18
investment, 7
irony, 101
isolation, 26
Israel, 92

issues, x, 10, 17, 22, 26, 33, 35, 40, 46, 50, 65, 73, 117, 118, 120, 121, 129, 150

J

Japan, 46, 74
Jewish Community, 92
Jo Roman, viii, 147, 150, 155
Jordan, 52
jumping, 27, 155
justification, 120

K

Kansas City Star, viii, ix, 112, 117, 127, 128, 129, 140, 143
kicks, 23
kidney, 82, 109, 116, 119, 120, 121
kill, 5, 6, 9, 12, 17, 23, 45, 63, 64, 150, 158, 163
Korea, 144

L

labeling, 25
laparoscopic surgery, 107, 115
latent content, 162
later life, 75
laws, 11, 139
layoffs, 128, 130
LDL, 109
lead, 4, 8, 24, 28, 46, 155
leaks, 51
learned helplessness, 21, 22
learning, 21, 68, 78
legal issues, 40
legislation, xi
life expectancy, 26
lifetime, 7, 18, 45
ligament, 108
light, 31, 119, 135, 140, 162
lithium, 26, 159
liver, 116
living arrangements, 35
local community, 28
local government, 27
Logic, vii, 11, 12, 13, 161
logical reasoning, 25
loneliness, 26, 40, 42
Louisiana, 75
love, 3, 5, 6, 12, 44, 65, 68, 69, 75, 89, 93, 95, 97, 101, 103, 104, 105, 123, 124, 128, 148
loyalty, 75
lying, 64, 78, 97